Holding On?

Hazel McHaffie
Ph D, SRN, RM

Books for Midwives Press
is a joint publishing venture
between The Royal College of Midwives and
Haigh & Hochland Publications Ltd

Published by Books for Midwives Press, 174a Ashley Road, Hale, Cheshire,
WA15 9SF, England

© 1994, Hazel McHaffie

First edition

ISBN 1-898507-21-X

British Library Cataloguing in Publication Data
A catalogue record for this book is available from the British Library

Printed in Great Britain by Cromwell Press Ltd

Cover photograph by:
Lionel F. Williams, Medical Photography, Royal Berkshire Hospital

Contents

Acknowledgements

Lesley Hobbs, Kenneth Boyd, Rosalyn McHaffie and Henry Hochland all influenced the production of this book. Their enthusiasm, encouragement and helpful comments are gratefully acknowledged. I am indebted to Libby MacRae for advice on the Scots idiom.

CHAPTER 1

Should he Live or Die?

'So, what it boils down to is this: do we pull out all the stops and keep Peter Flanaghan alive or do we allow him to die with a bit of dignity?'

Dr Roger Carshalton's voice sounded like the booming of a cannon in his own ears but was in reality barely above a murmur. A palpable silence descended on the assembled group as the enormity of the decision impinged on their thinking. For a fraction of a second, a wry smile fleeted across Roger's face as he weighed the balance of on the one hand this grave responsibility he carried and on the other the weight of the said Peter Flanaghan - all 597 grams of him. Here were nine grown people considering the potential of one scrap of humanity. And all before the infant had had any chance to show the world what he was made of.

It was Roger's registrar, Tom Faithful who broke the silence.

'Can we just check - the parents - where do they stand in all of this? Do they want us to continue treatment, d'you think, now they know - now they know how bad things are, I mean?'

'I think we've probably all got a slightly different view on this,' Roger replied, balancing his words carefully. 'Perhaps we could begin by sharing the messages we've each been given - or at least how we've interpreted what they've said - or not said, as the case may be.'

A few nods encouraged him to pursue this line of enquiry.

'Perhaps I could kick off and tell you what they seem to be saying to me. But of course, I do understand that as the consultant I'm perceived in a particular way and they'll probably have been more forthcoming with those of you who've had closer and more prolonged contact at the cotside.'

How hard it was to keep a proper balance. Roger knew he had to accept the responsibility that accompanied his position. The rest of the staff knew too. He was after all in clinical charge of this infant, ultimately answerable for any decision made on Peter's behalf. But on the other hand he had to give his colleagues freedom to voice their own beliefs and opinions. Roger assumed a brisker tone as he outlined his perceptions of the parents' views.

'Sue Flanaghan is I think genuinely desperate to have her baby live - whatever the consequences. She listens attentively when I try to spell out the costs in terms of Peter's prognosis and the suffering involved - for him, I mean, if we persist with this treatment. In fact she asks pertinent questions about what he'll be able to do. But when I mention the cost to her personally and to the rest of the family - the emotional and physical burdens - she seems to me to switch off and dismiss it as of no moment. I get a sense that she feels she has an unquestionable duty to care for Peter whatever his state or prognosis. It's simply not for discussion.'

'The Dad, Richard, gives rather different signals. He's very protective of his wife - quite excessively so, sometimes I think. On the surface, he seems to be coping extremely well - has done over the past three weeks since Peter was born - at least when I see him. Of course, I don't know what goes on away from here, but in front of me he's making all the right noises about supporting Sue, shouldering as much of the responsibility for things as he can. I get the feeling that he's keeping a fairly rigid guard over his own feelings when I'm talking to him. Tries to talk man to man - I don't know - almost as if we're discussing something quite unconnected with him.'

'I did actually set up a meeting with him on his own so that I could pitch things at the right level for him - perhaps give him a bit of support - but he didn't offer any insights into his own feelings. Kept the conversation at a fairly impersonal level as if we were both talking about this family we knew. He always came back to the mother's position and her needs - but it was as if he couldn't quite bring himself to register that it was his wife we were meaning. I have a sort of vague feeling that he's concerned about the burden Peter could become to Sue and that he's more prepared to consider an alternative to prolonging life, perhaps than she is.'

'D'you mean - he wants to let the baby die - so his wife isn't stressed?' Staff midwife Eileen Shorten spoke haltingly, fidgetting with her wedding ring as she voiced her question. Roger shrugged in response.

'I mean, what about him?' Eileen's brow puckered as she emphasised the 'him'. She shook her head, bewildered. 'What does he feel for the baby - himself?'

'I'm not sure - I mean, I really don't know. He doesn't give much away about himself - not to me.'

Turning from Eileen to the chaplain, Martin Lakes, Roger asked, 'What d'you think? Is he, perhaps, supressing his own feelings? I know the family has a strong religious affiliation, but I don't actually know if their church has a line on the sanctity of life. D'you know, Martin?'

Martin frowned in concentration as he contemplated the point of his pen before speaking. 'Well, Mr Flanaghan's a bit of an enigma to me too, I must confess. As you say, Dr Carshalton, he does - I don't know - he does seem to consider everything from the point of view of his wife. As far as his religious conviction goes, he just reiterates that, well, it's all in God's hands. But I really couldn't say whether he's prepared to give God a helping hand, or not. I did gently probe - very gently - to see whether he was in touch with his own minister. But I thought he clammed up a bit then. He just said - and he was quite short with me - he said the church knew about Peter. But I actually couldn't say if they've discussed the issues with their minister - or anyone else from the church - or not. He did actually say he'd appreciated the chance to talk about it with me. But it was a - I don't know - well, a polite comment, I suppose. More of a thank-you-for-another-pair-of-socks at Christmas time "thank you" - not a real, that-has-really-helped "thank you". And I didn't really feel we had discussed any of the important questions. But then, he didn't give me a sense that he wanted me to take the initiative there. I did gently introduce the subject of handicap, you know. Gently - tentatively, I suppose you'd say. But he just interrupted me, quite sharply. Suggested I keep them all in my prayers. I got the impression that he was basically saying - you get on with your job, keeping a line to God, and don't meddle in the rest of this business - not unkindly - don't get me wrong - but quite firmly, I'd say.'

'Well, I must say, I do think it's asking a bit much - expecting a man to bare his soul to an almost complete stranger when he's struggling to hold body and soul together!' The words came out with rather more passion that Catherine Woollard intended. As a senior sister in the Neonatal Unit she had seen so many families grappling with the horror of having a premature infant, struggling to survive in a world for which they were not nearly ready. How many parents had she consoled and supported. She saw the way they struggled too - struggled to retain some control. Precipitated into an alien world of machines, alarms, and bustling professionals, burdened by a sense of guilt that they were in some way to blame for this untimely birth, they felt so naked, so exposed. It was so hard to be surrounded by efficient but unknown doctors and nurses - when they met their infant for the first time; all during the days, the weeks, the months that followed. There was so rarely any moment of privacy in that highly charged atmosphere where everyone else seemed to have a role and a right to approach the baby but they felt so clumsy and fearful and so in the way.

'D'you feel you know him better, Catherine?' Roger's words were gentle.

'Well, not that well, I guess. But I do know that fathers, you know, fathers in general, they find it hard - hard to, well, share their deepest feelings in the Unit. Well, I think they have a pretty powerful need to be the strong ones, you know, there for their women folk. And, I think it's quite understandable - they aren't too keen to show their emotions in front of all the staff either. And another thing - I think it's hard for both parents to let go together. The fathers usually concentrate on supporting the mother at first - being strong and sort of taking it on the chin, themselves. They have their reaction later on when the mother's stabilised a bit more.'

'So d'you think Richard needs more time to assimilate the facts?' Roger probed.

'I'm not sure about that. It might take ages before he lets his guard slip. But - I don't know. That's not actually what I'm saying - at least, I don't think it is. I mean, I don't think that holding on to his - rigid control, would stop him being ready to, well, at least consider the arguments about how we deal with Peter. I'm only suggesting that perhaps we shouldn't expect him to - well - reveal his feelings about something so deeply personal - not to folk he's only just met, anyway.'

'Point taken.' Roger nodded as he spoke. 'Anyone like to suggest who might be able to get the Dad to discuss these issues?' His eyes moved from one to another of the assembled group.

He resisted the instinct to startle when the student representative on the group suddenly responded with, 'Would it be OK for me to try?'

Jo Manson was all too aware of her student status. But this was a subject about which she felt strongly. A qualified nurse of considerable experience, she had come at the age of 33 to train in neonatology. She had been in charge of a busy surgical ward when an accident has left her with a permanent back injury precluding her continuing in her post at her training hospital. With an inate desire to help others as strong today as when she had entered nursing as a bright young teenager, Jo had resisted any suggestion that she give up nursing for good. Infants were after all just as much in need of nursing care as adults but much lighter to lift. If she could move into neonatal care she might yet continue in the profession which was her life. Though relatively new to babies she was no stranger to family suffering.

She felt her colour rise as attention focused on her. But Roger's, 'You feel you'd like to have a go?' encouraged her.

'Well, I'm not sure I - want to exactly, but perhaps, mmm, perhaps I ought to. You see,' Jo took a deep breath, 'My sister had a prem baby 13 years ago. She - mmm, she nearly died herself when the baby was born - severe pre-eclampsia, you know. But even so, she insisted everything had to be done to save the baby. He did survive - poor kid. Very retarded. Doubly incontinent. Unable to even feed himself. My sister's partner, he couldn't cope with it all. He just left. Isn't even in touch. So there she is - having to look after Greg on her own basically. Just an occasional reprieve when one of the family goes in to let her away for a half day or so, so she can shop, get to the hairdresser, things like that. She's only in her thirties - tied, with absolutely no life of her own at all and no prospect of anything better either - which makes it all worse, you know, when there's no hope of any improvement.'

Silence descended again as the pain of this revelation permeated the listeners. It was Tom Faithful who broke into it.

'I'm sorry. I mean, I'm sorry to hear about your sister, of course. It's a ghastly tragedy when things go so wrong. But - what exactly would you want to convey, I mean to Richard Flanaghan, because of your experience with your nephew?'

'Ummmm, I suppose - I'd want to start off sympathising with him. You know, show him I know what it feels like, having something really dreadful happen to a baby. But then, I think I'd say it's important to think about what it means to the rest of the family too.'

'D'you think you might just be overly persuading him in one direction if you share your experience?' Tom pursued his point.

'No.' Jo's initial response was sharp as she felt a degree of resentment rise at the implication of the registrar's words. Already conscious of the temerity of her offer to intercede, she softened her retort with an explanation. 'I wouldn't just tell him what happened to my sister. That bit is just so he knows I know a bit what I'm talking about. I suppose I'd, I don't know, probably get him to talk about what it might mean to him, and to Mrs Flanaghan and to their little girl - in the future.'

'And what will you do when he asks you things like the probability of this or that disability?' Tom's face was impassive but his words conveyed to Jo his reservations about her suitability for this task.

Roger intervened swiftly feeling the hostility. Looking directly at Jo, he thanked her for her offer. 'It might well be very helpful for you to talk with Richard at some point - perhaps not just yet. And, of course, you wouldn't have to accept full responsibility for imparting information. We've all been trying to do that for several days and, well, I for one am not at all sure either of the parents are actually taking it in. An appeal to the emotions might just be the key.'

Turning then to the senior sister, he asked, 'Catherine, who would you say has had most contact with the parents? Who's got closest to them?'

Catherine hesitated a moment before replying slowly as she thought, 'On the medical side I'd say - Ira Ramshanshani. On the nursing side? Probably Wendy Greenaway and Eileen Shorten. I don't actually know how much social work have been involved. Have you had much contact, Harriet?'

As consultant in charge Roger knew all four and respected their contributions in the team. He realized with some dismay that he knew little about the views of any of them on the issues around prolonging life. It was something he must remedy. One of his obstetric colleagues had recently been reported by a nursing colleague - something to do with a late abortion. Difficult to sort out the truth from the fiction in these cases - they got so exaggerated in the telling. What the hospital did not need was another case of a member of staff blowing the whistle. Come to think of it, he didn't need it himself. Problems enough coping with the trauma and all the raw emotion without adding a court case.

Harriet Chase had been a social worker for 14 years but had only been involved in the Neonatal Unit for the last 18 months. She had a habit of nodding vigorously as each person spoke and sometimes gave an impression that she agreed with everyone. Now she nodded as she replied with, 'I've had, let me think, about three sessions with the parents. Really to find out about the home situation. The mother - well, she weeps quite a lot but she says they'll manage, don't need any help. She says Victoria, the other child in the family, is OK with her grandparents - you know, during this bit while they're spending so much time in the hospital. When I last spoke with her, she said Victoria was actually living with the grandparents - that's her mother and father. They're only about ten minutes away from them in the car.

'The father, now I find him rather prickly. He has this idea that there is, well, a stigma attached to having a social worker involved. OK, I know lots of them do! I've tried to present it as part of the whole package but I don't think he's really hearing that. He isn't very communicative with me and he certainly doesn't confide in me. So I can't really shed much light on this one, I'm afraid.'

'All right, thanks.' Roger turned from the social worker to the House Officer on his right. He was struck again by the striking good looks of the Asian girl with her thick, blue-black plait and liquid dark eyes. Ira Ramshanshani, in her turn, had developed an enormous respect for this compassionate man's approach. The life of a junior doctor on a busy Neonatal Unit was never easy and the long hours, demanding schedules and emotional load had more than once threatened to overwhelm her. She knew of colleagues elsewhere who had buckled under the harsh criticism of their consultants and was truly grateful for Roger Carshalton's understanding.

'Ira, Catherine thinks you are as close as any of us to this couple. What do you feel?'

'I have had quite a lot of contact, of course. We've discussed the prognosis and possible consequences quite frankly and I've always reinforced what you've passed on to me. But when I analyse these sessions - I suppose we've really always stayed with the facts. They ask me repeatedly how Peter's condition is and if there's any change. I try to give them as much detail as I think they can cope with. And of course I take my cue from their questions. On a couple of occasions when I felt I was getting out of my depth I suggested that they talk with you or Tom directly. I think they did pursue their point with you, Roger, but I'm not sure whether they sought out Tom directly?'

Ira looked across at Tom who shook his head briefly. Then she continued, 'Only once have I actually raised the matter of whether they'd ever want us to stop trying. It was Richard, the Dad, who instantly said they didn't want to talk about that. There was no question but that we should do what we could. Sue got in a bit of state, I remember. But she said she agreed and then started to weep again. I did wonder whether I should raise the matter with her on her own at another point but she hasn't given any indication that she would welcome such an opportunity. I am prepared to, if you think I should.'

'OK. Thanks, Ira. We'll come on to who will do what and when, a bit later I hope.' Roger smiled briefly at her before turning to Wendy Greenaway.

Wendy's thoughts were chaotic. It was several seconds before she began to speak. Ever since she had moved to the Alexandara Hospital in May of last year from a rival establishment 40 miles away, she had had an uneasy feeling that she was being watched. It felt like being on probation. And she wasn't yet fully accepted. They were watching - watching for those peculiar ways that showed she wasn't quite one of them - not yet. They didn't quite trust her to do things the 'Alexandra way'. When it came to the actual physical caregiving, on the whole she was confident. She had ten years of experience behind her after all. She could justify her methods. Most of the time she felt she passed the test.

But this - this was an altogether different matter. Her views on matters to do with life and death. They were nothing to do with where she had trained. They were something very deep, very personal and so dear to her that she was reluctant to expose them for public scrutiny. These new colleagues - would they understand how important they were to her? Better go cautiously.

She could stick to the Flanaghan family. That should be safe enough. After all, as Catherine had noticed, she had grown quite close to Sue and Richard Flanaghan. It was still so vivid, Peter's arrival. She had been on duty and it had fallen to her to lift the baby out of the portable incubator, unwrap him, weigh him, attach him to all the monitors. She remembered it now - the wonder she'd felt - always felt - at the perfection of these miniature babies. When his parents first came to see him, she had pointed out his perfectness. She so much wanted them to see that. Then the bad news, the set backs - they wouldn't take them quite so hard. Not if they saw the perfection first.

When she's told them and they knew - really knew - they'd produced something very wonderful, then she could tell them about all the routines which must now characterise their trips to the nursery. It hadn't been so hard to explain the equipment swallowing up their baby - the Flanaghan's were calm, intelligent, articulate people. They listened, they understood. Not like some of the parents - the hysterical ones, the angry ones, the poorly educated ones. And it had been a special moment - that third visit when she had encouraged Sue to reach into the incubator and touch the stick thin arm for the very first time. Sue had cried and she had had tears in her own eyes too. Just the sheer emotion of that experience for the mother. A special bond had been forged between them all.

Taking a deep breath now, she lifted her head higher. Pushing her curly hair behind both ears, she began to speak, her low musical voice betraying her Welsh background.

'I agree with you, Roger, the husband's very protective of his wife. They've had a bit of an unhappy life, one way and another. I expect you know - but perhaps not everyone does? - apparently, they adopted a little girl several years ago and she drowned in an accident in a relative's pond. Ghastly, isn't it? Richard told me about it one evening. He actually said he feared for Sue's mental state after that and he says, he just doesn't know what would happen if she lost another child.'

'Yes, it was Richard who told me too,' Roger interjected.

'Sue herself - when I talked to her about the tragedy - she said Richard was marvellous at that time and she can't speak too highly of his support. But, I'm not sure, reading between the lines, I think - I think she still grieves terribly for that child but I also think she feels Richard expects her to be over it, so she can't really talk to him about how badly she feels. She told me - in confidence - that she frequently goes to the grave and sits there for hours and hours sometimes. But she says no-one else knows she does that. So please, everybody, don't mention that to her or anyone else. She leaves Victoria with her parents and pretends to be going shopping or to see friends. But she actually goes out to the grave. Richard is immersed in his work as a teacher and Sue feels because his days are so packed with other demands and interests that it's easier for him to forget. Could very well be.'

Wendy paused for a moment as a tap at the door heralded a call for the chaplain saying that he was wanted in Ward 17. Martin Lakes hesitated.

He rose and excusing himself left the room with a muttered, 'I'll see if I can transfer the call to Keith Richardson'. As the door closed behind him, Roger turned back to Wendy.

'Do go on, please.'

'I don't very often see Richard without his wife but on a couple of occasions quite near the beginning, he actually popped back in to be with Peter on his own after he'd taken Sue back to her bed at night. I don't quite know how to explain it, but he seemed quite a different person then. When Sue's there he stays back, lets her touch the baby, change him, and so on. I did ask him once if he'd like to reach in and hold Peter's hand too. But he just shook his head, said something about his hands being too big and clumsy. But then, when he was there on his own, he moved in, you know, really close to the incubator, whispered to the baby for ages hardly taking his eyes off him. It felt sort of - well, sacred time somehow, so I moved away as much as possible to give him space and privacy. So I don't know what he was whispering.'

She paused remembering the electric air of that encounter.

'And the other time?' Roger prompted.

'The second time, off his own bat he opened the porthole, reached in, stroked Peter's arm and put his finger into Peter's hand so that his little fingers curled round it - you know, like they do - and I saw a tear drip on to the incubator. But I haven't been there when it's just been Richard on his own - not since then. When he comes with Sue he seems sort of switched off to emotion. He looks at Sue as much as at Peter - always making sure she's comfortable, got what she needs and everything. Although it sounds sort of special and loving, I don't know. I can't quite put my finger on it. But it doesn't feel quite right somehow. It's - I don't know - oppressive? No, not exactly oppressive. I suppose - it's a bit - a bit too intense, yeeees, yeees, that's it, I think - it's too intense when you'd expect him to be more concerned about Peter. But then I remember those times when he was on his own with the baby and I'd say he does love the baby too and is grieving for him. Just, when Sue's there he can't seem to see beyond her. I'm not expressing this very well. Sorry.'

'You're doing fine.'

'But it's not easy to define exactly why it doesn't feel quite right. He talks to me and is pleasant and friendly enough - well, they both are. Nice couple. Usually once they've asked how the baby's doing and looked at his charts and things they talk about other things - like Richard's school day, Victoria's antics and sometimes ask about my outside life.'

'You mean you have a life outside these sacred portals?' Ira quipped and a small ripple of laughter relieved the tension momentarily.

Wendy responded with a twinkle but otherwise continued in the same calm reflective way as if simultaneously recalling and analysing what she had observed.

'There is one other curious thing I should mention but I really don't know what it means. Once - must have been when Peter was about a week old - the parents were both sitting beside the incubator when Richard's parents came in to see the baby. He seemed to me to be ultra polite with them - you know, as courteous as you would be with strangers. But there was - I don't know - there didn't seem to be any warmth, any - you know - familiarity, somehow. Sue seemed relaxed with them but not Richard. It might be nothing but it just felt odd. I don't know if anyone else has noticed anything?' Her eyes scanned her colleagues but no one spoke and several shook their heads.

Self deprecatingly she commented, 'Maybe I imagined it then.'

'No, it's useful to hear your sense of what's happening as well as what you actually observe,' Roger reassured her.

'As far as their feelings about Peter's future go - I can only say, they both seem to me to be pretty desperate to have him live. Neither of them has asked me anything about stopping treatment but they do quite often ask about what the damage to his lungs and to his brain means - you know, in real terms. Yes, both of them ask those sorts of questions - the same questions over and over, of course, but we expect that, don't we? Parents in these sort of situations usually do. I haven't raised the subject of taking him off the ventilator and letting him die, of course.'

'Of course?' Roger quietly questioned her rationale.

'Well, I have very strong views myself about that and anyway it's not really my place to.' Roger noticed the tightening of her lips and made a mental note to ask her privately what those strong views were. It would be wrong to force a declaration in public.

'You've obviously got quite close to this couple to learn so much about them. I'm sure we all appreciate that insight. Thank you for sharing that with us, Wendy.' A warm smile in her direction accompanied Roger's thanks. 'It goes without saying that any confidences shared in this group remain here and I know we will all tread sensitively here. OK, over to you Eileen.'

'I have to say, I haven't seen anything odd with the grandparents although I don't personally take to Richard's mother. Yuck!! But perhaps I shouldn't say that!' Eileen clapped a hand to her mouth, blushing a little at the indiscretion. She felt rather relieved when Ira and Wendy nodded vigorously with rather sheepish looks on their faces. 'Oh, that's a relief. You feel the same. It seems sort of mean to say it when you know they're having to cope with some pretty traumatic experiences. I'm not quite sure what it is, but that Granny seems quite oppressive I find. Even when she comes on her own with her husband and the parents aren't there, she seems to adopt a sort of hectoring tone. I get a feeling she's constantly on the look out for something to complain about. Her husband, he seems a rather meek kind of a guy. He never meets your eye when you're talking and he seems really uncomfortable all the time - fidgeting around. And he never asks a question; never begins a conversation. It's quite hard going relating to him. But Granny Flanaghan, ughh, she makes me feel like I am about to be caught out in a misdemeanour!'

They all smiled at this matronly figure portrayed as a naughty schoolgirl. For Eileen Shorten, a part-time member of staff, had a wealth of experience with neonates and of life in general behind her. The mother of five children herself, she had retained a zest for this work which many envied. Her maturity coupled with her lively sense of fun made her a popular figure in the nursery and she was in receipt of many a confidence when her juniors needed advice. Now, with her ample roundness settled in a low slung chair she looked like an amiable grandmother. For her to feel chastened seemed incongruous. Smiling in response to their amusement, Eileen went on.

'The other grandparents, they're really nice. Really gentle souls and they're so grateful for all that modern medicine offers for Peter. Hoping desperately that he won't be horribly handicapped - and praying for a miracle.

'The parents? Well, I think Sue's a bit like her mother. Devoutly hoping for a miracle. She seems to want to concentrate on the facts and figures about the ones that do well in spite of the odds stacked against them.'

Eileen saw heads nodding in recognition of Sue's propensity to focus only on the positive.

'Sue's never mentioned the child that died - not to me. But I knew about it - from Richard right near the beginning. He said she couldn't cope with losing another child. I agree with Wendy, he doesn't talk about his own feelings. All he seems to worry about is Sue. But it's quite nice really - in a way - the way he sort of cherishes her. He seems to want to protect her from life somehow. But I guess lots of women'd give their eye teeth to have a chap like Richard cherishing them like that. Maybe I'm just jealous!'

Those who knew her husband, Bob, smiled at her comments. They knew how good he was to Eileen.

'Do you feel Sue accepts his protection?' Roger was listening intently.

'Well, I must say, on the surface she seems to. She certainly speaks warmly of how good he is to her. I suppose I do wonder if they do actually talk about the problems together - on an equal level, if you know what I mean. If it came to deciding whether to continue to battle for little Peter, I'm not sure if Sue'd be given the space to say how she feels. But I could be quite wrong.'

'We should have to make sure we gave her that space,' Roger interjected.

'Well, I wasn't meaning, you know, physical space. Would she - I don't know how to put it - would she know how to deal with it on her own, without her husband speaking for her - p'rhaps even thinking for her - if she's fallen into the pattern of letting him always take charge? If, you know, like Wendy says, she's grieving secretly for the other little girl - you know, the one that died - does that mean that she can't let Richard know how she's really feeling about other things? I don't know, but we perhaps ought to know'.

Roger nodded his head, looking down at the notepad in his lap. After a brief check that Eileen had finished her statement, he summarised the position as he saw it.

'I accept what you're all saying and what I'm hearing, I think, so far, is that we as a team haven't really got the measure of this family fully. We feel that there are undercurrents which we can't really explain. But we need to fathom them better if we're to approach the Mum and Dad on the very delicate matter of Peter's treatment - whether we continue heroic measures or whether we let him die with dignity. I have to say, I don't think we are quite at that point yet. We do have other avenues still to pursue with the baby but I feel, perhaps we should start preparing ourselves for the possibility. Does anyone want to say anything else about the family before we move on to other interested parties?'

At this point the chaplain re-entered the room with apologies as he slipped back into his vacated chair.

'Time and tide ...' he whispered to Harriet with a grin.

Roger courteously gave him a resume of the proceedings so far before moving on to the issue of the staff's own feelings about this child's future. Here he knew he was on treacherous ground. There were a number of unknown elements in the group and he was aware of how difficult it was in the frenetic pace of this high powered unit to properly get to know how his colleagues felt about things. In spite of sharing so many emotional situations with them, you only really saw the professional fronts. Was it self defence that made each keep something of themselves from the scrutiny of others? Was he too remote in his seniority? After fourteen years as a consultant neonatologist he knew that feelings ran deep and strong on these matters. Simply being with a baby for hours on end tending to his every need, developing a relationship with each member of the family, made these caring people fiercely protective of their charges. Added to that, he was all too conscious of the weight of strong religious convictions, of personal agendas, of life's experiences. He felt he could probably guess at the reactions of Tom Faithful who had been his registrar for three years now. The most senior member of the nursing team, Catherine Woollard, he had worked with for even longer and she had discussed these things with him on various occasions similar to this one.

The chaplain made no secret of his beliefs and Roger welcomed his forthright declarations leaving everyone in no doubt about where he drew his own ethical boundaries. The position of the remainder of the group was largely unknown to Roger and he felt the unseen presence of the rest of the Unit workforce. What a task it was to make such momentous decisions when so many others relied on him for information and wisdom. And yet they were all in a position to report him if his decision flouted their idea of the ethical norm or accepted standard of practice. All right for them, they didn't have to accept the final decision - they could say their piece and walk away. He had to live with the consequences for the rest of his life. Frightening how caring cooperative sensible parents and staff could change to venomous litigacious critics when things went wrong.

CHAPTER 2

Whose Decision?

Roger took in the serious faces, the unease, as he outlined the problem. He had to go cautiously if these people were to declare their own personal views on Peter's future management.

'I know we're all a bit tense when we start to think and talk about prolonging life and allowing babies to die. We've all seen enough of the cases which have come to court, to know we certainly don't want to be blazoned over the front pages of the tabloids. These issues I know affect some of us in particular very deeply. Some have strong religious beliefs. Others have had particular personal experiences that influence how we react. It's OK to have such views and I'm sure we shall all respect each other's position. But we're a team. We have to work together on this. I think we must be careful not to be overly persuaded by the most passionate arguments - they're important but then so are the ones that are calm and reasoned.

'You will all recognize that I have to take the final decision but I'm a firm believer in the team approach. If you all feel very differently we won't of course be able to please everybody. But it would be good if we could discuss the issues openly and arrive at some kind of point where we could all accept the decision and the reasons for it. We've seen quite clearly how the parents relate to each of us slightly differently. And it's been really helpful to hear how you all perceive them. So could we try to share how we each feel ourselves about the future for little Peter?'

Although no-one spoke Roger felt their acceptance in principle.

'For the benefit of those of you who're not intimately involved in Peter's clinical care - Martin, Harriet, anyway - would it help just to briefly explain Peter's condition?'

'Mmmm, please,' Martin nodded. Harriet just kept on nodding.

'Because he was born so prematurely his systems are very immature and he's toiling. First of all, he has collossal breathing problems. He's been ventilated since birth to help his breathing and he's still on maximum oxygenation. Even with that his lungs are in pretty poor shape and that's in spite of the surfactant therapy which should have helped to lubricate his air passages. Surfactant? - you know ...?'

They both nodded again, familiar with the name of this drug.

'Basically he just can't get enough oxygen for his needs by using his lungs. In real terms that means it's unlikely we shall wean him off of oxygen for a very long time. He's horribly susceptible to chest infections - he's had several courses of antibiotics already. On top of that he has a Grade 4 ventricular haemorrhage. From the scans we think he's suffered major brain damage from the bleeding into his brain and he'll be pretty severely handicapped if he does pull through. So as you'll appreciate the little chap is in quite a mess.'

Roger noted the dismay in their faces.

'I think we have to do two things here. We have to consider how we individually, and as a group, feel about withdrawing treatment in general and we have to consider how we feel about continuing Peter's treatment in particular. Once again, can I stress - what's said here is confidential. I don't want anyone to feel, "Oh I can't say that! What if someone reported me" or "What would they think of me if I told them that's what I believe!" I'm sure we all recognize that there's a huge spectrum of thinking on these matters. There aren't too many absolutes. We all need to respect each other's position. So, fire away.'

The long pause was slightly disconcerting but understandable and Roger forced himself to sit still allowing them space.

It was Tom who volunteered the first comment.

'Well, I might as well come clean. I don't believe in God so I don't have a problem with this "playing God" bit. And in any case I don't see that stopping treatment is any more playing God than starting it in the first place. It does bug me that some of these kids are going through hell from the treatments. I mean, the ventilation, the chest drains, the physio, the heel stabs, pretty well everything we do to the little beggars. Well, it must be hellish. They can't tell us how painful it is. If they dare to fight the ventilator we paralyse them so they can't move but they must still be feeling it - they just can't protest!'

Tom's rather rough manner seemed oddly at variance with the sentiments he was expressing and more than one person looked their surprise. In general he was seen to be a rather cold operator who did the job but didn't get involved. More than one nurse had smarted from his withering dismissal of their views and a rather abrasive tone inhibited colleagues from getting to know him better as a person.

'Well, we aren't as barbaric as we were a few years ago. We do at least use analgesics now.' Roger retorted. 'Not like it was when we even operated on them without drugs.' Out of the corner of his eye he saw Harriet Chase wince and her face contort at the thought.

'OK, I accept that, it is better - but I'm not convinced it's enough. We are all so damned cagey about being taken to court because we've given too much morphine or whatever and put the little perishers out of their misery.' Tom sounded almost belligerent. 'These folk who see it all, say nothing but then go blabbing to the press or the Pro-Lifers or whatever - they've got a lot to answer for.'

Inwardly Roger's heart sank. This was not the way to get the doubters to open up. The lowered eyes and uncomfortable movements betrayed the barriers were being raised.

'It's exactly because we don't want to have this kind of unpleasantness dividing us, that we're having this discussion,' he said. 'I have to confess, I personally sympathise with anyone who has a real difficulty with discontinuing treatment. It's tough. If you've been looking after one of these little sproggets for weeks, got really attached to them, it tears your heart to see them die. If other people who don't seem as involved, so attached, are making the decision and you have no opportunity to say how you feel about it, it's even tougher.'

Silence again allowed the group space to think. It was the chaplain who spoke next.

'I come from quite a different place from Dr Faithful. I do believe in God, it won't surprise you to hear!' A smile greeted this statement. 'I accept,

OK, any intervention is in a way "playing God", but I have more of a problem with stopping treatment than with starting it. I suppose for me, my sticking point comes in relation to the handicapped. Are we saying the value of the life of a handicapped child is in some way less than that of a "normal" one?' His fingers traced the apostrophes as he spoke. 'I mean, if Peter Flanaghan would be normal in the end, would we try harder or for longer? I can't help feeling that if you asked handicapped people if they'd rather live with all their problems or rather not exist, mostly they'd choose to live. And I have to say, although it seems callous when you articulate it, they haven't actually known anything else so they aren't comparing a life of problems and pain with a "normal" life.'

'Would we try harder if Peter was otherwise normal?' Roger repeated the question thoughtfully. ' I think my personal response would be, I want to see the size of the odds stacked against this little chap. His chances of survival are pretty slim anyway. But let's say he does pull through against our predictions. In all likelihood he'll be blind, spastic, paralysed, incapable of forming a relationship of any real quality with anyone else, totally dependent on others for the whole of his life. We're not talking about a cheerful little chap in a wheelchair who can feed himself, go places, be educated, appreciate the love of his family, the companionship of his sister, the friendship of the world. Disregarding the burden on his family for the moment, I'm not personally totally persuaded that it's in his own best interests to have a life of pain and suffering without any compensating benefits. But of course, I know some people think all life is sacred and I respect their point of view too. In many ways I rather envy them their position - it's a view that you can hold to more consistently than mine. Mine depends on circumstances and forces me to make judgements about best interests and rights.' Roger was doing his best to give everyone permission to speak up about their divergent views.

'I've already said I have strong views about the sanctity of life so I might as well own up to what they are.' Wendy's head was held high and only a slight flush on her cheeks betrayed her apprehension. 'I'm a Catholic and I do subscribe to the belief that all life is sacred. I admit, I do. But that doesn't mean I go about reporting my colleagues!' she added defensively. 'My heart goes out to the families having to shoulder these ghastly never-ending burdens and I wouldn't want to force my opinions on them. Not at all. But I couldn't personally be any part of the process if you do decide Peter isn't to be treated. I'd be sad about that. I feel I've got quite close to the parents - and to Peter - but my conscience wouldn't let me be party to allowing him to die when we have the means to keep him alive. I guess it will sound soppy to the rest of you, but I also think these tragic cases can bring out finer qualities in the folk who care for them. OK, I accept, Peter might not be aware of much that's going on around him. But caring for him, loving him, could make Sue and Richard finer people. Is that the word I'm looking for? But you know what I mean. I know personally I feel good caring for someone who can do nothing for me in return. And well, I don't know, even in really severe cases, carers get satisfaction from tiny things - things that seem to us very small rewards. Things like, well, a grunt or a finger moving that seem to show the disabled person is responding - that can keep them going for ages.'

'Aahhh, but what about all those families where the child drives wedges between the rest of the family? Their lives are ruined. You can't say that's bringing out the best in them!' Jo's eyes blazed as she almost spat the words out.

Remembering Jo's nephew, Wendy nodded. 'I know. I know. It doesn't always work out. But I suppose I feel - well, I wonder - can we tell which families will be strengthened and which will disintegrate under the strain? I don't think we can if we don't give them a chance.'

'So you'd make them all go through with it and tough on the ones that go to pieces?'

'No, I'm not saying that ...'

'Well, you sound to me as if you are! Excuse me!' Jo interrupted.

'I didn't mean to imply that. I think it matters what the parents are prepared to cope with and to accept. But, if they can't face dealing with the consequences, to me - and I'm only stating my personal belief - the answer's not then - eliminate the cause of the trouble - the child.'

'So what d'you do then?'

'Well, I think you try to find an alternative source of caring.' Wendy saw the sneering look that came over Jo's face, but she continued, trying to keep her voice calm and not betray the stress she felt from the other woman's aggressive tone. 'Something like - I don't know - foster parents or somebody. After all, it isn't the child's fault that they've been born with all these problems. It's not their fault if the family's not equal to the challenge. So what gives us the right to bop them off?' Wendy felt so strongly about this issue that, in spite of her dislike of contention, her voice rang with confidence.

Jo was obviously rattled. 'Well, I must say, no disrespect to you personally, Sister Greenaway, that doesn't gel with the world I know! My sister can't get even basic help with Greg. No matter how depressed, how exhausted she gets. The services just are not there to give her - people like her - a break. They offered her a fortnight in the summer - you know, what they call "respite care" - once. So she could go off on holiday. "Recharge her batteries" the woman said to her. OK - seemed like a good idea. But when she got back ...' Jo paused remembering.

Shaking her head at the recollection she went on, 'Greg was so much more difficult - like he felt he'd been deserted, you know, and was taking it out on her. And his skin was in really bad shape and Val, she really works hard to keep his skin intact, free from infection. It's something she feels very strongly about. She was heartbroken - heartbroken to see the state he was in - after only two weeks. Made her feel no-one else was to be trusted to look after him. So all in all things were so much worse after the break, she wished she'd never gone away. She's never done it again.' Abruptly her tone changed from sad to militant as she voiced her sense of the injustice of her sister's plight. 'Oh, it's OK if you get cancer or something respectable like that. Then you can get Marie Curie nurses. You can have someone staying the whole night. All sorts of help. But have a multiply handicapped kid and you're on your own, matey!'

Wendy opened her mouth to respond but Jo was in full flight by this time, anger overtaking her natural reticence. 'And as for this idea there are foster homes and foster mothers queuing up to take care of these kids - forget it! I simply don't believe there are those folk around who'll care endlessly for other people's abnormal kids - well, maybe there's the odd one here and there. But certainly not enough to take on all the babies we'd have on our hands if we kept all these damaged kids alive. And we all know about the raw deal they get in institutions!'

'OK.' Roger's interruption was deliberate. His tone was quiet after the passionate exchange they had just witnessed. 'I think we'd all accept that things are far from ideal. But sometimes we have to aim for the ideal if we are to reach a 'good enough' level of care - given all the constraints we are grappling with all the time. I'd like, if I may, at this point to return to something Wendy said earlier - about not being party to the process. I understand what you're saying. And of course we don't expect anyone to do anything against their conscience. Can we suppose for a moment that we do decide the right thing to do is to discontinue treatment - only supposing. We haven't decided anything really. OK the majority decision then is to withdraw treatment. Is it a problem if someone else disconnects the equipment say, and there is the time when Peter needs to be cared for between then and his death? Would your position be that you wouldn't feel you could help the family then?'

'Well, I'd be really torn, I must admit. I know I'd have a lot of anger inside me at what had been done. I couldn't help feeling that because of how much this all means to me.'

'OK, we understand that.'

'I wouldn't blow the whistle but I think - yes, I think I'd feel a sort of lack of loyalty in a way to some of my colleagues. It'd be difficult - it'd be very difficult to answer the parents' questions. I couldn't - I mean, I couldn't reassure them that everything was being done that could be done. Or that it was best this way. Not if I didn't think it was. But I would be torn. My instinct as a nurse, as a caring human being, would make me want to stay with them, until the end - to support them, be there with them sharing the agony and everything but there would be a real conflict of interests. Practically that would make things very awkward.'

'Thanks. I respect your point of view there and of course, there would be no suggestion that you would be opting out of a painful task. I'm sure we've all seen you in operation sufficiently often not to doubt your integrity or compassion.' Wendy felt a surge of gratitude for Roger's sensitive response. 'But, of course, the family would be the poorer for your withdrawal. Now, what does everyone else think? Please do contribute - we need to get a sense of the general feeling as well as the specific objections or support or whatever. We are hearing so far that personal beliefs, religious convictions, the interests and rights of the child, the quality of life he could expect, and the resources of the family might all influence how we deal with this case.' He ticked each item off on his fingers as he listed them.

Ira had felt unusually troubled by the tension between Wendy and Jo's conflicting views. Now she began hesitantly. 'I must say, I'm terribly glad the buck doesn't stop with me on this one. I think I'll specialise in pathology!' Roger grinned, glad of her lighter touch. 'I don't know how relevant this is, but I think it probably matters how closely we're involved. That perhaps influences how we react. I don't know. The nursing staff especially get very close to these babies and to the Mums and Dads. We tend to breeze in and breeze out again and we're dealing with all sorts of other things so these isolated specially painful cases, stay in a wider context. But you,' her gesture embraced the four nurses, 'You're shut in these rooms with this baby - and the relatives - for whole days together. I imagine it would be much more agonising to lose the baby then. A bit of you must die too sometimes and I suspect you're mourning in a deeper way than us a lot of the time. Not that we don't feel it too, I don't mean that. But I think it might be to a different degree. So, what I'm leading up to is, I think that you should speak up, all of you, because this isn't just about rehearsing the arguments for and against prolonging a life. It's about how we can manage these things - practically. And what it means to us individually. And I think you're nearer to how the parents are feeling than probably I am anyway, I can't speak for Tom or Roger. But they're of age and can speak for themselves!' Again her flash of humour lightened the mood of the assembled people.

Ira sat back to allow the nurses to speak. In the ensuing pause she reflected on the situation in this Unit compared with others she knew of. Roger was trusted by them all, she felt sure of that. No Dracula here going about with a lethal dose of something in his pocket. He really cared about these babies. And their parents. She'd personally be perfectly happy to leave Roger and the Flanaghans to work out a solution. But it wasn't fashionable to talk about paternalism these days, she was well aware of that. Anyway other people did seem to want to have their say. And of course, if they didn't get it, Roger could be open to more public criticism, perhaps even legal action if somebody got a bee in their bonnet about things. She wouldn't wish that on him.

But there again, she probably felt pretty laid back about it because she didn't have strong feelings about the absolute sanctity of life. She actually felt very reluctant to hand on a burden to parents which she wouldn't want to carry herself. Wendy now - she seemed like an intensely caring sort of girl - she probably would be the self-sacrificing kind.

'Well, while we're all waiting, can I say something? As Ira says, I am of age and I can speak for myself.' Tom's tone belied the light reference to Ira's quotation. 'OK the nurses are probably closer to the parents than we are but I do have a problem with them wanting to make the decisions. After all, it's our,' he tapped his chest with one finger, 'our medical defence subscriptions that go up and up. We're the ones who end up in court - not the nurses.' Why oh why did Tom have to be so provocative, Roger wondered.

Catherine felt she had to intervene now her profession was in the firing line and in any case her seniority dictated that she should respond on behalf of her team. Inwardly her hackles were up but outwardly she sounded calmly reasonable.

'I don't believe the nurses are wanting to make the decisions actually. But having said that, they do have a contribution to make to the debate. They are, Ira's just said it, usually closer to the families. In eight or more hours continuous contact with a baby on each shift you get to know all sorts of things about them, things that single them out as real little individuals. And after all, if a decision's made that the baby is to be allowed to die we are the ones who sit with the parents - help them cope with it all - well usually. I know Roger's more than once done that himself and the parents have been really grateful.'

By way of explanation Roger chipped in. 'Those were occasions when I felt the last stages were too painful to ask someone else to do it. Not when I'd made the final decision that it was better to let the child die. But anyway, in general terms, I think it's actually rather important not to forget how bad it feels. I don't know if it's possible to get glib about life but I don't want to get to that stage if I can help it.' He made a gesture to Catherine to continue.

'That's it really, I think. I don't think nurses do want to make the decisions. But having said that, we do appreciate opportunities like this one to be able to say how we feel. And of course, in our defence I can say, we are accountable for our own practice, so if things definitely aren't right in our judgement then we are obliged to speak out. If there aren't these team meetings where we can discuss particular cases openly together, it will drive people to report colleagues - just simply because they can't live with the consequences of other people's actions.'

Although her response had been in reply to Tom's comment Catherine studiously avoided meeting his eye as she spoke. For some reason she had never liked him. It was not just his withering comments about the nurses but something in his manner which made her freeze inside. She dreaded Unit rounds when he was in charge - he seemed to imply criticism in all sorts of ways and made everyone nervous or upset.

'Thanks, Catherine.' Roger turned to Eileen and raised his eyebrows to invite her to speak without putting her on the spot if she didn't want to contribute at this point.

Eileen came quickly to the support of her nursing colleague. 'I agree entirely with Catherine. We don't want to make the decision. Actually I think I'd go so far as to say, I'm pretty sure most of us are devoutly thankful we don't have to. But I agree we can supply information to round out the picture. And of course we do have beliefs and moral positions of our own. We're entitled to have those! My own position is definitely coloured by a personal experience we had in our family - what, about two years ago now. My father was terminally ill with liver cancer and bone secondaries. He was in agony. He knew he was dying. He begged my mother - begged her - to leave his tablets near his bed so that he could take the whole bottle. She just couldn't bring herself to do it. Then Dad asked the GP, Dr Blackstone - he'd been a family friend for years - he asked him if he would put him out of his misery. He was very sympathetic. But of course he said he couldn't - he couldn't do that because it was against the law. But he listened really attentively, said he'd try even harder to crack the pain. Well, in fairness, Dr Blackstone consulted the experts at the local Hospice; he tried several different cocktails of drugs. He did his best. And I'm not blaming him for refusing to ... well, to do what Dad wanted.

'But Dad still just wanted to be finished with all the pain and indignity. He wanted to die at home too. Actually he was really resistant to going in anywhere even temporarily. I think he was afraid if he went in he'd never come out again. He wouldn't even go into the hospice to see what they could do to relieve his symptoms. That was what I wanted him to do. I may as well tell you, he asked me to do it too - give him a fatal injection, I mean. Said I had access to drugs and would know how much to give and everything. But I just couldn't do it. Not because I thought it was wrong. I wouldn't let Stephanie's hamster go through suffering like that! But I couldn't risk it - couldn't risk the legal action that might have come, you know, afterwards. It would have killed my mother. And anyway I think she'd never quite have trusted me again. She didn't see it like I did. She just didn't want to lose him. And it would probably have finished me career-wise too - and we need the money my job brings in.

'Anyway, my Dad asked my brother to leave enough tablets near him so he could do it himself and that's what Jim did. One day when he went to get a new prescription he just put them in the bedside cabinet. Dad took the lot that night.'

A long pause enabled Eileen to choke back the tears as she remembered the pain of his death. Her voice trembled as she continued her story.

'I was really angry - really, really angry - when Jim told me. Not because he'd given Dad the tablets - oh no, I admired his courage in doing that. I knew how much he loved Dad. But he should have told me - then I could have said goodbye. I never had that chance. If he'd told me I could have gone - knowing it was for the last time. We live a long way away from my Mum and Dad - well, Mum now. I'd been going down about every fortnight but it was costing us a packet. With all the children needing things, ferrying them around and everything there just wasn't the time to be always there - even if we could afford it. But the last time I saw Dad I'd had to tell him again I couldn't just kill him off. He was just so angry - accused me of just not caring what his life was like. I mean, deep down I knew he was only mad because he was in such pain. But I hated being out of favour like that. And I never saw him again. So we couldn't make it right like it used to be. Jim should have told me.'

Eileen's voice trailed away as tears overtook her control. Catherine reached out to lay a hand on her arm and Eileen blew her nose fiercely. Used as they were to displays of grief in the Unit it was still discomfiting to have a colleague so distressed. But a warmth of support flowed out to Eileen as they sat quietly waiting for her to compose herself.

Roger felt the onus was on him to steer her into stating her position in relation to Peter. She would later regret her revelation if it had not fulfilled its rightful purpose.

'Has this experience changed how you feel about prolonging life, Eileen?' he questioned gently.

'Well.' Again a vigorous noseblow helped Eileen regain control of her voice. 'I always thought perhaps there was a place for helping people out of a totally awful position. I mean, I used to think it would always be possible to find a mixture of analgesics that could control the pain but I know from what I've read and from what I've seen and from Dad's experience that it isn't always possible. Even a walloping dose doesn't necessarily do the trick. But it's not just the pain. I mean, Dad, he was a fearfully independent character and a very private man and well, he just hated - hated, the indignity of the whole business. I think it's quite hard for us to appreciate'. The sweep of her hand took in the entire group.

'I mean, we get so used to seeing ill people in various stages of undress, not in control of bodily functions, all of that. But when you're a man like my Dad - never had much to do with hospitals - well, what we do to them - it's a diabolical liberty! Sorry, I forget what I was supposed to be talking about.'

She turned to Roger with a rather sheepish look and a questioning incline of her head.

'Your views on prolonging life?'

'Oh, yes, thanks. Sorry about that. I get a bit carried away when I get on to this subject. Well, what I mean is, I don't think we should be deciding for our patients and their families. They're the ones who have to live with this ghastly situation. We can walk away and go and do our own thing. They live, breathe, sleep, eat it! So my view is - once we know that medically there is nothing more we can do and the outcome is grim, we should let the family decide how they want it to go.'

'That was a very powerful contribution. Thanks, thanks a lot, Eileen. I'm sure we all appreciate what it costs to talk about something so deeply painful. But I wonder what you'd think, say, if the family don't all see it the same way. OK, in your father's case he was the principal sufferer and you knew what his wishes were. But your mother and brother and you all had a slightly different opinion.'

'Well, not exactly,' Eileen interrupted. 'I wanted to take the same line as Jim but I couldn't because of my circumstances and really I suppose because I knew too much about the consequences. Jim didn't really understand the legal aspect - he couldn't see beyond Dad's suffering.'

'OK.'

'As it happened, there were no questions asked about Dad's death. He was so near the end anyway with being absolutely riddled with cancer that they expected him to go at any minute. Dr Blackstone didn't even suspect anything, I don't think. He didn't ask any questions. Just signed the certificate. And we didn't have to have a post mortem so Jim got away with it, so to speak. I can say this here because it's confidential and anyway none of you know where my family live so you couldn't do much about it. Anyway I don't believe any of you would be mean enough to do anything like that.' Her frank tearstained look defied them all.

'OK. So you and Jim felt the same but your mother didn't approve. In the case of Peter, we haven't pursued this issue in detail with the parents but if, say, we suspect that Mum - Sue - wants Peter to live at all costs, but Richard can't cope with the burden on Sue and suppose he says discontinue treatment. Some of us are a bit concerned about relationships with the grandparents and suspect something is going on there. We already have a difference of opinion amongst the professional staff. How do we proceed then, would you say?' Eileen looked intently at Roger as he spoke, mentally schooling herself to put her father's death aside and concentrate on the issue occupying the minds of these colleagues.

'Well, it's easy to just give a pat answer, I know. But, of course, I do know it isn't easy - well, we all do, don't we? Especially when parents are terribly emotionally frazzled. But, well, I suppose I think - I think you'd have to speak to them each alone - try to get at what they really feel. Then perhaps bring them together and discuss things generally with them both, giving them the facts and probabilities as far as you can. Then, if they present a different picture when they're together, I think you'd have to introduce in a gentle sort of way what they had disclosed in private.'

'Except that you might be losing their trust by doing that - if they told you how they really feel - in confidence. Don't you think?' Roger asked. 'For example, if Sue tells me that while there's life there's hope and that she is utterly opposed to stopping treatment but she'll be guided by Richard - because he always makes the important decisions. Then let's say, when I see them together, Richard does all the talking and he says, stop the treatment. And say, Sue just agrees with him. If I then tell Richard what Sue really thinks, I could be seen to be betraying her confidence. She might have a lot of problems with her relationship with Richard as well as not trusting me any more.' Roger's eyes were still on Eileen inviting her to expand on her ideas.

Eileen nodded agreement. 'I accept that. But if you don't get the communication lines open now that kind of situation between a couple -

the mixed messages, suppressed beliefs, unshared wishes - can fester and cause untold damage later. It might be better to let some of the anger and hurt be hung on the doctor - someone a bit removed - rather than have it all directed at each other.' She grimaced as she suddenly realized the burden she was so easily handing to someone else.

Roger smiled and gestured with his hands to show he accepted her point.

'Anyway, if they're going to have to live with a severely handicapped child or live with the knowledge that they are sort of responsible for him dying, then I'd say, the odds are against their relationship surviving intact from the outset. I know it's a very delicate balance. But I'm sure - 'cos they've known you throughout and 'cos they respect you for your real compassion towards Peter - they'll understand you're only trying to do what's best for everyone in all of this.'

'So, if I can summarise, you think the decision should be the parents' once we arrive at a point where we think further medical treatment is futile. And I should try to get a consensus view from them. Is that a fair assessment?' Roger asked.

'Yes, I think so. It sounds sort of bald put so succinctly but, yes, that's about the size of it.'

'I wonder if I can come back to something rather more fundamental?' It was the chaplain who moved the discussion on. He had long toyed with the philosophical arguments relating to prolonging life and assisting death and was fascinated by this debate which brought those issues into stark relief because they were focused on a living sentient being, one of God's own creatures.

'In a way I think all medicine's a form of divine intervention. I mean, just stopping people dying of pneumonia or appendicitis is a sort of 'playing God'. But I'm sure none of us would advocate letting nature take its course at this level. Then, medicine has got more and more sophisticated and we - or perhaps I should say, you - have got cleverer and cleverer at saving babies. I mean, about - what - 20 years ago, Peter wouldn't have stood the remotest chance of surviving and we'd have consigned him to the mortality statistics with a touch of regret but no real discussion about it. My point is, isn't stopping the treatment or allowing him to die - or assisting him to die - simply an extension of this progress? Medicine has produced this phenomenon of a tiny baby on the very edge of viability actually breathing on his own. Isn't it just an admission that we aren't really in a position to go further - given present knowledge. And maybe we should now withdraw? I don't know. I'm open to persuasion but it doesn't feel like something so heinous to me to withdraw treatment when, on mature reflection, you all recognize that it isn't really working for this fellow.'

'I accept your point, Martin, but I think what it boils down to is what isn't "working" in Peter's case. OK, we are extremely doubtful about his survival. So, if he simply doesn't make it in spite of our best efforts then the problem's solved for us at least. It didn't "work". On the other hand, he might keep fighting and surprise us all. If he does we think he will almost certainly be severely damaged. In that case, something is "working" after a fashion even though the consequences are fearful. He is after all alive. So what is it we want to "work"?' Roger's question was addressed to the whole group.

'I like your analysis of the state of play, Martin,' Ira Ramshanshani broke in. 'I hadn't really thought of it in those terms before. I suppose the sticking point is that people regard life as something so sacred that once it's in being they don't think we have the right to dispose of it.'

'Except that that's exactly what is being done thousands of times every year in this country alone with legalized abortion!' Jo Manson interrupted.

'So perhaps that's where the difficulty arises,' Martin continued meditatively. 'The law hasn't really been able to deal with this so it remains a thorny issue. So it's difficult for us to resolve.'

'You're dead right there!' Tom's words came out with strong feeling. 'The law's definitely an ass when it comes to differentiating between forms of killing. It twists my guts to see fellow medics hauled through the courts accused of murder when they've simply been trying to do their jobs and relieve suffering. These damned lawyers seem to take a perverse delight in outsmarting the doctors with their clever words and innuendos - trying to trap them into saying things they don't mean. "Answer the question, Doctor, yes or no!" Tom mimicked in a falsetto voice. 'How many of them have sat and agonised over what the right thing to do is when you've got all these people's lives to juggle with? I guess they get so used to dealing with the criminal classes and waging their stupid battles with their fellow legal eagles that they don't really care who is innocent and who is guilty. It's just about, "How many cases have you won this week, Sebastian?"'

The listening colleagues smiled ruefully at Tom's outburst sympathising with his passion.

'I'm sure we all know what you mean, Tom,' Roger soothed. 'And of course you are absolutely right - the law doesn't differentiate between cold blooded killing and the sort of compassionate ending of a life of misery we're concerned with. Having said that, I don't think we are talking about taking active steps to end Peter's life, are we? I think we are trying to decide whether we think it's appropriate to withdraw aggressive treatment and allow him to die peacefully and probably surrounded by his parents' loving arms rather than isolated in the incubator attached to miles of tubes and machinery. I, personally, certainly hadn't anything more dramatic in mind. The position seems to me to be narrowing down a bit. If he doesn't survive in spite of our best efforts, there can, I imagine, be no criticism of our management. So, I think we're down to one question really. Is this little chap's potential quality of life and its consequences on his family justification for allowing him to die sooner rather than later?'

'So, is it a question of how sacred is life? Or how bad does a life have to be not to be worth living?' Martin asked.

Roger thought about the question for a long moment before he replied. 'Both, I suppose. In fact, I think they are both aspects of the same issue, aren't they?'

After a brief pause he turned to the social worker. 'From the point of view of the family's coping resources, how would you rate their ability to cope with a severely handicapped child supposing together they and we decided it would be right to continue to treat Peter? Are they reasonably competent to deal with such a burden, would you say from your experience of such families?'

Nodding steadily, Harriet replied, 'It's always difficult to say with any certainty. Until people are in that situation even they don't know how much they can take. But with what I've seen so far, they are reasonably comfortably off so they could probably manage without Mum having to work. They've a house which they own - well, they are buying it, mortgages and so on, you know. And they live in a reasonably affluent area and own a car so they're mobile. I haven't seen inside the house of course, but there shouldn't be a problem with space, I wouldn't think. As far as personal resources go, well, I really don't know. The nurses probably see more of that side than I do. But I suppose the fact that they are in a stable relationship and seem to cope well with Victoria - she's a cute little thing and seems very well behaved - seems to indicate they are adequate parents. They do have both sets of grandparents within hailing distance and certainly the Mathieson grandparents seem to have a lot to do with Victoria - I guess they might be a source of support. I have no idea how they'd respond to a handicapped child, of course. It bothers me to hear about Mrs Flanaghan's reaction to the death of the other little girl. I didn't know about that. It does make you wonder if she could cope any better with the chronic sorrow of having a disabled child. I've seen very together families crack under the strain of the endless work and drain.'

'OK, so materially fairly well endowed but some of us are anxious about Mum's coping ability.'

'Excuse me, but are we to consign a child to death just because his mother isn't as robust as we'd like her to be?' Wendy's indignation was apparent.

'I don't think anyone is ready to consign anyone to anything as yet,' Roger replied quietly. 'All we're trying to do is get as fair a picture of the family as we can at this stage so we can assess how best to go forward.' He was acutely aware of the daggered look Jo darted at Wendy and not wishing to exacerbate a potentially volatile situation he decided it was time to round off the meeting.

'Time's gone, I'm afraid, so we must draw this particular meeting to a close. I know we haven't exhausted the subject yet. Thank you all very much for your helpful contributions to this discussion. I think I have a fair picture of where we are with this. As I've said, I don't think we are quite at the stage of making this momentous decision but it's been helpful to discuss it at this point - I'm sure you'll all give it further thought. If things develop and we get to a point where discontinuing treatment is a definite option, I shall hope to have further discussion with some of you anyway. I realize there are other people out there in the Unit who may well have strong views and I'd be grateful if you could each let your own circle of folk know that they'd be very welcome if they want to come and discuss this case with me. It's obviously not going to be possible to include everyone in these team meetings but Catherine and I have tried to get together those of you who have been most closely involved with Peter and his parents.

'I plan to be around for the rest of this week, no conferences or anything scheduled, so I should be accessible. In the meantime I shall, of course, be meeting with the Flanaghans as before and keeping close tabs on Peter's progress. You'll probably like to know that I've had lengthy discussion with my consultant colleagues, Adrienne Tamworth and Bill Forsyth, and I should expect to involve them in any final decision. If any of you want to make any further contributions, please don't hesitate to make contact with me and I'll do my best to make sure everyone gets a full and fair hearing. I'm sorry to break it off here but I know that three of you at least have other deadlines to meet and the glances at the timepieces have not gone unnoticed! Thanks, everyone.'

It had been a powerful meeting and Roger was desperate to get away and down some strong black coffee. Instead he slipped out of the room and went to look at Peter Flanaghan lying so still, paralysed with pancuronium to stop him fighting the ventilator. How laboured his breathing was. Poor beggar. Little did he know that his whole future existence had been in debate this morning. The staff nurse responsible for him on this shift reported the current ventilator settings and blood gases and Roger sighed shaking his head at the picture.

'Mum and Dad around today?'

'They were in first thing and Mum is planning to return straight after lunch. She's very weepy today,' Carol Elmslie replied.

'Could you let me know when she comes in, please? I'd like to see her.'

Yes, he definitely needed a strong coffee.

CHAPTER 3

Mother to Five

Eileen Shorten's heart sank as she opened the gate and walked towards her front door. The sound of heavy metal music rocking the very fabric of the building meant that Victoria was home and drowning out everything in her life that grieved and irritated her. Eileen had sometimes stood a silent observer in the doorway watching her painfully thin seventeen-year-old gyrating, convulsing, succumbing to the pounding of the beat, eyes tightly screwed up, every muscle taut as she lost herself to all but her innermost thoughts. She had always been a very tense child but puberty had exaggerated her inclinations and she had retreated into a world from which her parents were definitely excluded most of the time. It was only when she reached a point of utter desolation that her veneer cracked and she became the little girl in need of solace. Then Eileen could satisfy her maternal longing to wrap this tortured creature in her arms and rock her as she sobbed out her fears and insecurities. At all other times the mother knew she had to respect the five feet of private space Vicky had thrown around her person.

Today Eileen was not ready to assume her maternal mantle; her own wounds were too raw from that Unit meeting. In the first place, she identified herself far too closely with Peter Flanaghan's parents. How could one make such an appalling choice? And why, oh why had she exposed her own feelings like that? What did they all think of her now? Why hadn't she just kept her mouth shut?

As well as that, all the way home she'd been feeling annoyed - well, perhaps not annoyed - disappointed in herself - yes,that was it, disappointed. Because she had ignored the needs of others - a thing she rarely did. She had always had a big heart - always been ready to listen and help other people, no matter how trivial the problem. And today she had turned away from people - her colleagues - her friends - when they probably needed somebody to turn to. She just hadn't had anything left to give. Talking about her Dad like that, her own pain and everything - she was wrung out. Empty.

So when she heard the raised voices in the changing room, she'd hesitated for a fraction of a second and then turned on her heel and gone back into the nursery. She'd heard enough to know the hint of hostility they'd witnessed in the Unit meeting had escalated into a direct confrontation. The tone of Jo Manson's voice - the blistering dismissal of Wendy's cherished beliefs - had frozen her in her tracks. Her first thought was for Wendy - quiet, caring, a superb neonatal nurse. Must be so hurtful to have your convictions scorned in that harsh way. But Jo too, she was hurting - hurting enough to attack a senior member of staff. Strange girl, Jo. She seemed such a cold character. Kept herself to herself. Efficient but not much feeling, Eileen had thought. Maybe she had feelings that went too deep for words. Even though she hated confrontations herself, she found herself strangely moved by the passion behind Jo's ferocity. It must be profoundly troubling to have a severely handicapped child in the family - even if he was only a nephew.

By the time she arrived home she had quite convinced herself that she had let her colleagues down badly. Always so quick to blame herself. Silly, she knew, but she couldn't help it. Tomorrow she'd feel stronger. Tomorrow - tomorrow she'd do something about it - whatever 'it' was. Now all she wanted was to crawl into a corner, bury herself in a warm cocoon, and let the tears flow. But the small uncomplicated body of her five year old, Stephanie, flinging damp clinging arms around her legs in a rapturous welcome, even before she had closed the door behind her, put paid to any such indulgence.

'Hello, poppet!' Her arms scooped up the little creature sweeping her higher until their eyes were level. 'How've you got on today?'

'Mummy, Mummy, Mummy.' The arms squeezed tighter with each repeat. Then with her face buried in her mother's shoulder, she blurted out her news, her lisp more pronounced than usual in her anxiety. 'I've been ever so naughty, Mummy. Vicky says so.' She lifted her head and peered closely into Eileen's face trying to read her reaction to this confession.

'What have you done?' Eileen's tone was exaggeratedly solemn even while inwardly the youngster's expression tickled her desire to laugh aloud.

'I - I - went into Vicky and Rachel's room, an' ... an' ... an' ...' Her confidence tailed off as she heard Victoria descending the stairs four at a leap. Again the arms tightened around her mother's neck.

'Oh, you're home.' How cold Vicky seemed at times. Eileen hugged her baby daughter closer wanting to keep these soft warm arms around her shutting out the hurtful things.

When Vicky had whirled into the kitchen, she turned back to the moist grey eyes at her shoulder.

'What did you do in the girl's room, poppet?'

Stephanie took heart from the smile and the endearment.

'Well, you know Vicky's black lipstick? You know?'

'Uh huh.'

'Well, I was only lookin' - first, Mummy. Then - then - then I tried it - just a lickle, tiny, weeny bit, Mummy. Only a tiny, tiny bit.' The podgy fingers showed how infinitesimal the crime. 'Only I couldn' - I couldn' - get it straight - not like Vicky does. Vicky gets it straight. So then - then I used a cloth - it was on the dressin' table by the lipstick - it was on'y a cloth. And I rubbed it off so it - so's I had it on, like Vicky does - you know, Mummy. Like Vicky does. But she came in - and she was very cross Mummy - crosser'n you, Mummy, when I'm naughty.'

The bottom lip trembled and a slow tear welled and fell with a spreading darkness on Eileen's blue shirt.

'She said - it wasn' a cloth - it was her new shirt. Bu', Mummy, it was on'y a lickle, lickle cloth. I didn' know it was a shirt! I didn' mean to spoil it - hones', I didn' mean to.'

Eileen hugged her close, soothing the pain of rejection whilst reinforcing the house rules on privacy.

'And did you tell Vicky you were sorry?'

'Yeh, yeh.' The vigorous nodding dislodged the last tear and the tumbled dark curls danced about the blotched face.

The black whirlwind that was Vicky in full motion reappeared but this time her mother blocked her passage.

'Vicky, Steph has told me about the shirt. Can I help to repair the damage?'
'Nope.' Vicky made to move on but Eileen remained blocking her exit.

'Is it that bad?'

'Nope, I've washed it myself and it'll be all right.'

'Well, it would've been a kindness to let Steph know, wouldn't it? Instead of leaving her to stew - thinking she'd committed some cardinal sin?'

'She shouldn've been in my room! She's nothing but a pest!'

Eileen felt the head burrow into her neck as Stephanie heard but couldn't comprehend the reason for her sister's vitriol.

'She knows she shouldn't and we've gone over all that again, but you could be a bit more gracious about her apology, couldn't you? She has feelings as well as you, you know.' Didn't they all! But Eileen recognized with a sigh the rebellious turn of her eldest daughter's lip and without another word moved aside to let her pass into her own world of dark self-centredness.

Five children had turned Eileen from a crisp, efficient almost fanatically tidy person into a rounder, more dishevelled woman constantly compromising her own tendencies and wishes to meet the ever-changing whims and vagaries of her family. This was definitely the most trying point of her day. Returning from work, not yet having shed the inevitable emotional baggage her demanding job brought with it, she craved a period of quiet to unwind before adopting the multifaceted roles of parenting such a motley band of children. Instead she was always precipitated instantly into the thick of all their joys and pains. It could be just as much of an effort to listen to a tumbled catalogue of the events of a happy day as to decide on the merits of two combatants in a squabble over who had the right to choose the TV programme tonight. Any demands on her attention were superfluous to her own personal requirements. Peace and quiet her body and brain demanded. Peace and quiet she could never find.

She had never really been able to reconcile the competing demands of motherhood and paid employment. Ambitious she was not but she loved her work and knew that this outside dimension made her a more interesting and less intense mother. She could never have coped with Vicky and Rachel's moods if she had been home all day with nothing more stimulating to keep things in perspective. But she so often wondered if she was neglecting the younger ones. She couldn't always be there for them, not with the varying shifts she was required to work. Night duty had been a useful stopgap but the eternal sleep deficit had affected her health and she had been obliged to change to day shifts. So everyone had had to take on some responsibility for the running of the house. Visitors looked in amazement at the neat rotas in the kitchen, bathroom and hall. Did children really do things like dusting and hoovering in these modern times? The Shorten children certainly did. Not always with a good grace but there was no question about whether you did those chores. This was one area where you could never play Mum against Dad.

Still clutching the remorseful Stephanie in her arms, Eileen moved wearily through to the kitchen. A cup of tea might help to improve the complexion of the evening. No sooner was the kettle filled than two muddy forms erupted through the back door. Timothy and Nicholas were still young enough to be instantly pleased to see her. Their game of football had expended vast wadges of energy and they were temporarily stilled as they flopped into chairs around the scratched wooden table, the scene of so many family conferences. Dragging his grey soggy socks on escaping tired feet, Timothy went to the fridge in search of a drink for his younger brother and himself. They were good friends, these two, caught in the middle of a triangle of girls. A rough camaraderie sheltered them from the unfathomable complexities of their older sisters changed by emerging womanhood from the pals they used to be. Their boisterous interests distanced them from Stephanie but she, with her undemanding love and admiration for them, brought out a gentleness in the lads which warmed Eileen's heart. As he returned to the table and plonked the lemonade in front of Nick, Tim tousled Stephanie's curls and asked nonchalantly, 'Hi, pumpkin, wan' a drink?' The smallest offspring brightened at his interest and nodded her head rapidly.

'Yes, please.' Eileen's correction was automatic.

As the three drank noisily she poured her tea and joined them in a rare moment of verbal silence. The warm liquid soothed her frayed feelings and she soaked in the unconscious acceptance of her which these three youngest children exuded.

'What time's Dad home?' Nicholas didn't even look up from his absorption in his glass.

'About 6 - he hopes.' Eileen glanced at the clock. Forty minutes to get on with the meal before he was scheduled. 'Who's turn for veggies?'

'Mine,' Tim replied instantly, 'But can I just go an' have a shower first, Mum? My shorts're dead muddy an' my feet're freezing!' As he spoke he rose from the chair, ear ready tilted for her response. Eileen saw the soggy wetness on the chair and felt his discomfort even as she granted permission and moved to get a cleaning cloth before some other unsuspecting person sank on to the booby trapped seat.

He was gone in a trail of squelchy footsteps and a faint aroma of male sweat. Nicholas began idly walking his fingers across the table towards his sister and suddenly tickling her under the chin. Her giggles and scrunched up shoulders relieved the last of Eileen's tension about the incident with the shirt. How she envied this ability to obliterate a pain as soon as it was confessed.

'You'd better get into something dry, too, Nick,' Eileen said, looking briefly at her younger son's mud spattered football strip. 'In fact - gather up both lots of muddy gear and stick them in the machine before tea - would you, please?'

'Yep.' He rose from his seat scraping the chair harshly on the tiled floor.

'And what about homework?' Her question was casual as she began to assemble the ingredients she needed to tonight's macaroni cheese.

'History. Gotta look up 'bout Napoleon.'

'OK. Don't leave it too late getting that done, then.'

'Nope.' Nicholas slouched clumsily out of the kitchen. Finding herself without a playmate, Stephanie began to pound the table rhythmically with the flat of her hand. Eileen's nerves were too frayed for any such innocent irritation today. But, skilled in diplomacy after so many years of practice, she offered a task of grating cheese and breadcrumbs which made the small face sparkle. Much better to have the energies usefully diverted even if she would pay the price of so much more mess to clear up at the end of the operation.

Once she had set up her daughter's field of activity to ensure maximum safety, Eileen suggested, 'Let's play a game. Let's see who can go longest without saying a single, single word!'

'Yeeessss!' This was one of Stephanie's favourite games and Eileen felt a twinge of guilt at her double motives for introducing it.

'OK. Starting ... now!'

Peace descended. It was so calming to have nothing more to distract her than the sauce making. The sound of the macaroni bubbling over on to the hot ring made Stephanie grin conspiratorially at her but she kept her lips tightly compressed in her effort to still her recalcitrant tongue.

When a transformed Tim bounced into the kitchen, Stephanie waved her arms to attract his attention before putting her finger to her pursed lips to show him what was afoot. He, too, knew the rules and entering into the spirit of the moment began gesticulating exaggeratedly to his mother to ask which vegetables he was to prepare. She pretended not to understand his question for a few moments before producing a bag of carrots and small basket of peas she had picked that morning. Tim settled himself at the table and set to work on the peas as silence again descended.

The savoury dish was golden and crackling under the grill by the time Bob got in from work. One look at his face and Eileen knew he had had a tough day. He had been a fireman since she had first met him 21 years ago and she had learned to live with the effect of his traumatic experiences. At first she had felt hurt by his closed reaction that excluded everyone, including her, from his private hell. The mother in her wanted to share his hurt and soothe away the pain. If she didn't understand the nature of the trouble she couldn't help. But gradually she had come to accept that there were some things that went too deep for disclosure. He had to escape from her probing; forced revelations would merely add to his burdens. He simply couldn't let himself dwell on the horror - the charred bodies of children trapped in an upstairs room, screams stifled as they suffocated before the firemen could reach them. The motorway carnage that left six people dead, mutilated beyond recognition. The agony of staying with a young cyclist - a lad of Tim's age - as he lay trapped beneath an articulated lorry that had jack-knifed on that cruel bend on the A1.

It was Stephanie who, in her innocence, did what he most needed. As soon as he appeared in the doorway of the kitchen she forgot her determination to beat her mother in their silent game and hurtling across the room, she shrieked, 'Daddy! Daddy! Daddy! See what Mummy and me's made for you!'

Bob caught her up in his arms and hugged her close as he followed her pointing finger. The macaroni cheese did indeed look good and he was sincere in his fulsome praise. A quick squeeze of his wife's waist and the arm as soon withdrawn told her without words his control was fragile and she responded with a brisk, 'Good timing! It's just ready. Can you give the kids a yell while I serve?' A good yell was just what he needed but his restrained summons of the other four children had to suffice.

For both Eileen and Bob there was an artificial air to this meal. Aware of their internal turmoil, they were yet glad of the outward normality and trivialness of this family gathering. Correcting table manners, hearing about the daily events from the younger childen who were still not too much upon their dignity to share their lives, they could take comfort from this sanctuary where nothing seemed more important than Rachel's exam tomorrow or Timothy's clean bill of health at the dentist this morning. Out there the world could be a cruel hard place. Within the warmth of this steamy fragrant room, they wanted to wrap their children up and protect them from life's darker side.

With the wide age range from Vicky to Stephanie bedtime was a much protracted affair. Bob had elected to read to his youngest daughter tonight and had been gone such a long time that Eileen went to investigate. She found him, fast asleep in the chair, one arm still curled around an unconscious Stephanie, his greying head nestled beside her damp black curls, the book sliding from his grasp as he let go of the tensions that held him so fast. She stood for a long moment looking down at these two dear people. Then, dropping a kiss on the soft cheek of her baby, she stole from the room, closing the door to protect her husband from the intrusion of the older children's noise. She envied him his ability to fall asleep so easily. When she was stressed she often got to a point where her mind would not let her body get the repose it needed.

The evening hours were all spoken for in Eileen's timetable tonight. Nick was in the school play and she simply must get on with his costume. What Mrs Trevelyan thought she could do to present him as a bush, she wasn't entirely sure. She knew only too well her younger son had no artistic or dramatic ability but he was inordinately proud of being included in the school production. She owed it to him to make him the finest bush that had ever graced the stages of Europe! So she applied herself with more vigour than real enthusiasm to the task of cutting out hundreds of green leather and vinyl leaves.

The boring repetitiveness of her actions produced a rather soporific effect and she was pleasantly switched off to anything but her cutting when the shrill ringing of the phone beside her broke her trance. She groaned inwardly as her mother's querulous voice asked how she was. It was sure to be a long listen so Eileen propped the phone between her shoulder and ear and continued plying her template and scissors. Tonight though half attention would not suffice. Her mother was soon in tears and Eileen had to exercise all her skill and sensitivity to discover what had happened. There had been a leak in the roof and the man who had come to mend it had told her she needed a lot of other things fixed and she couldn't afford it and what was a poor widow woman to do all on her own? Eileen wanted to know if her brother knew about this, after all Jim lived only 20 minutes away in the car. Well, he did but you couldn't expect him to drop everything and come to sort out her problems. After all, he had such a high-powered job. Eileen resisted the impulse to catalogue her own commitments and concentrated on soothing her mother before she talked through the best course of action. Throughout this long conversation the boys had been alternately watching television and playing a rather boisterous game of Twister, which involved them twining their bodies into impossible positions and collapsing in fits of hysterical laughter. It was very hard to hear above the noise of their hilarity, but Eileen felt so guilty shushing them. In the end she found she had agreed to travel the 200 miles this coming weekend to see what she could do. Bob would definitely not be pleased. He had promised himself a weekend to get the small bedroom painted.

It was tough being a woman at her stage in life, Eileen mused. You were caught between the competing demands of three generations and whichever way you went you were sure to be wrong. It was 40 minutes later when she could finally put the phone down and her voice was unexpectedly sharp as she roared at the boys to be quiet and get ready for bed. Why couldn't Bob be there and sort them out? Sheepishly eyeing her heavy frown, Tim and Nick slunk from the room unable to suppress the instinct to punch each other in a friendly sort of way as they jostled at the bottom of the stairs.

A window-rattling crash from upstairs indicated something was not as it should be. Since the boys were still in sight, it had to be Rachel or Vicky - or both, this time. Whose idea was it to have five children? She arrived precipitately in their room only to find her oh-so-sophisticated daughters taking flying leaps from one bed to another attemping to somersault on the floor space in between. Given their wild appearances, clad from head to foot in unbroken black, faces caked in pasty white make-up and their hair standing in a state of suspended animation from a too liberal application of gel and hairspray, they looked like Macbeth's witches in mid-incantation. The teenagers had the grace to look crestfallen as their mother stood, hands on her hips, with tightly compressed lips surveying the scene of devastation they called their room. Through gritted teeth she instructed them to grow up and consider other people for a change. Sullen looks descended and the abandoned enjoyment of a moment ago was lost. Eileen was past Freudian analysis. She was beside herself with tiredness and had no more reserves for wayward daughters. They had half an hour to re-establish order! Did order ever exist in this convoluted world of teenage standards?

'But, Mum!' Rachel wailed, 'I haven't finished my homework yet!'

'You should have thought of that before you decided to clown around and ruin everyone else's evening!' Deep down Eileen knew she was exaggerating their crime out of all proportion but she could take no more - the tension had to go somewhere.

'I have to get my physics done tonight! The Old Phantom'll kill me if I'm late with it again!'

'Again?' Her mother's voice was icy.

'Well, I forgot it last week.'

'How do you **forget** homework?' Eileen had always tried to instil a sound approach to hard work and responsibility into her children. Sometimes she wondered it these two girls were suffering from wierd mutations in their chromosomes, they seemed so alien to her.

Rachel knew when she had pushed her luck to its limits and she backtracked a degree or two. Adopting a more conciliatory tone, she coaxed, 'If we get on and get this mess cleared up, can I have just one more hour to do my Physics - **please**, Mum? I promise I'll really get on and I'll be ever so quiet ... **please**?'

With a resigned sigh, Eileen gave in, redeeming her reputation in her own eyes by delivering a strict admonition to make it one hour and not one minute longer. Her reward came.

'Thanks, Mum - you're an angel!'

Instantly the two black skinny figures set to work and Eileen left them to their wierd rituals. Would Rachel become as complicated to deal with in a couple of years as her older sister, she wondered? At least there was still some way of appealing to her at the moment and she did seem to recognize that her parents were entitled to discipline her. Vicky was another kettle of fish altogether.

Almost as soon as Eileen had settled back down to her cutting, the sound of the bathroom door closing and a scampering of feet across the landing followed by a dull thud indicated that Nick had finally made it to bed. Once again she wearily climbed the stairs, ignoring the muffled giggles from the girls' room, and went in to bid her younger son goodnight. Warm arms enveloped her neck as he nuzzled against her bent head.

'Mmmmmm, you smell nice, Mum. Thanks for the scrummy macaroni cheese. It's my most favouritest thing in all the world! Is it OK if Ben comes to tea tomorrow before we go to Scouts?'. She returned his embrace with interest, smiling at the jumble of his thought processes. The last thing she needed right now was another mouth to feed, another body filling the crowded space, another set of feet to trail mud across the carpet but she responded warmly with her usual, 'Of course, darling. And thank you for appreciating the meal. It makes it all worthwhile when you remember to say thank you for it. Another of your favourites tomorrow - fish pie!'

'You are the bestest Mum in all the world - and I 'spect in the whole universe! How bigger'n the world is the universe, Mum?'

'Bigger than I've got time to tell you now! Night night, sweet dreams!' Eileen always loved that moment when she looked down at the children's heads on the pillow - so trusting and innocent. She knew what people meant when they said the early years were your best. But growing up had its compensations. She enjoyed the more serious discussions she could have with the older girls - when they were in a mood to treat her as a person and not too preoccupied with establishing their own infinite superiority.

Popping her head round the door of the sitting room to remind Tim that he had only another ten minutes, she finally returned to her leaves. She liked working in the kitchen on the big table, surrounded by the comfortable sounds of the old Railway station clock and the kettle simmering on the Aga. The soul of the house was here and she liked the constant toing and froing of the family keeping her in touch with their activities as they called in for drinks or comfort. When Vicky wandered in in an apparently accidental way half an hour later, Eileen greeted her with, 'D'you fancy a cuppa? I'm having one if you want to join me.'

Vicky agreed and instantly offered to make it so that her mother could get on.

'Don't you get fed up having to do all these things for all us kids, Mum?'

'Not usually. Only when I'm dead beat,' her mother replied with a smile. 'Why? Do I seem fed up?'

'Not specially, only I'd hate to have to always be doing things for heaps of other people. I'm not gonna have any kids.' Her heavy emphasis on the 'any' made her mother smile.

'There are an awful lot of nice things about having children,' Eileen reviewed her feelings during the past hour rather ruefully. 'And when I see the problems some Mums have at work I feel very thankful with my lot!'

'What kinds of problems?' Vicky was busy with mugs and teabags, but her mother sensed one of her rare moments of communication.

'Well, we've got a very sad case at the moment. We've got a tiny little fellow in - he doesn't look good. If he does make it he's going to be horribly disabled. And the Mum and Dad might have to decide - any day now, - whether they want us to keep fighting for him or whether he ought to be allowed to die - with a bit of dignity instead of wired up - tubes in all directions - machines doing everything for him. I'd hate to have to make that kind of choice if it was one of you children.' The scissors were still and Eileen's gaze went way past her daughter as she reentered the painful world she had left a few hours ago.

Vicky passed her the steaming mug and watched her mother take a sip before she asked, 'What would you do - if you were her, I mean?'

'What would I do? Ahhhhh. I think - I think I'd say I wanted them to stop the treatment now. We've given him a chance - hasn't really worked. It's been a sort of - I don't know - a sort of trial of life, you know? See if he can hold his own. And I don't think this is him holding his own. If I were his Mum, what I'd want would be to take away all those tubes and everything, wrap him up in a special shawl I'd made for him myself, take him out of the incubator. I'd want to sit in a big rocking chair - like I used to do with all of you when I got up to see to you in the night. I'd cradle him in my arms an' love him an' kiss him an' everything - hold him till he died. I'd want to put a whole life time of loving into that little while - an' I wouldn't want to put him down or let anyone else touch him or take care of him - nobody else - just me.' Eileen seemed almost unaware of her daughter's presence as she felt the intensity of those precious minutes, every one representing years.

'Is that what she'll do?'

'I've actually no idea what she'll do, poor soul. It's going to be heartbreaking whatever she decides. Thank God I've never had to lose a child - can't even begin to think how horrendous that would be. Till you've had a child you just can't imagine how much you'll love them - it's something - something so big, so special, so - so wonderful - you can't express it.'

'Is it bigger than how you loved Dad when you were in love with him - you know, at first?'

Eileen knew how her daughter's mind was working. She had recently fallen desperately in love with Craig, a rather lanky lad with poor eyesight and two left feet but a wonderful smile that clearly transformed him into a veritable Adonis. She would die without him!

'Oh, it's quite, quite different. It's something to do with the baby being - part of you - and being so utterly dependent on you - and being so - so wonderfully made and - oh, I can't really put it into words. But being a Mum is the most fantastic thing I've ever done - and I thought it with all five of you. And even when we have our bad times,' they exchanged wry smiles, 'I still love you all - more than I can ever really tell you. But you know that, really.'

'Well, I'm glad you're my Mum an' you're a real Mum.' Vicky's emphasis on the 'real' warmed her mother's heart. 'Lots of the kids at school have

Mums who don't seem to want to be Mums at all. You're a sort of home person. Like the Aga in the kitchen. You're the sort of Aga in our family.'

'What a lovely thing to say.' Eileen was deeply touched by this compliment from her currently most distant daughter.

'But I'm not an Aga person so I'm not going to have kids!'

Eileen let the comment pass and instead said, 'The Mum - the one I've been telling you about - she has a daughter called Victoria but she never calls her Vicky.' They both grinned remembering a phase in her life when Vicky had refused to answer to the abbreviation. 'Makes me feel I can identify with her - specially, you know?'

'Can you have a say in what happens to that baby, Mum?'

'Well, we had a meeting about him today actually.'

'And?' Vicky was impatient with her mother's pausing.

'And we could each say how we felt.'

'What did you say?'

'I told them about Grandpa and how I thought we ought to let the family decide because they have to live with the consequences, not us.'

'Gosh, that's awesome!'

'How do you mean?' Eileen was startled by her response.

'Well, I thought - you know - when you're at work, well, you're Nurse Shorten an' you didn't talk about the family. I mean you don't tell them about - us - do you?' Vicky's expression betrayed the nightmare this possibility conjured up for her.

Eileen laughed. 'Sometimes I do - in conversations with my friends - of course, I do. You're part of my life!'

'Well, I hope you don't tell them the bad things.'

'Some things are just too horrible to repeat! Seriously though - actually I've been feeling badly about talking about Grandpa and Grandma and Uncle Jim this morning at the meeting.'

'Why?'

'Well, because I was nervous, you know, about speaking in front of everybody, I got a bit upset - not weeping or anything serious, but I was a bit tearful, you know - remembering Grandpa and everything. I wanted to stay very cool and rational. But they could see I found it hard to talk about and I expect my sentences were all jumbled because I was flustered and, I don't know, I probably made a fool of myself.'

'I'm sure you didn't. Any case, I'd take more notice of somebody who knew what it felt like - you know, more'n somebody who just made a good argument. When Grandpa died, there was this girl at school I hardly knew, an' the day I went back to school, afterwards, you know, I was really afraid I might start to cry. So I was making myself be really busy and stuff an' trying not to think about Grandpa an' the funeral an' everything. An' anyway this girl came up to me an' said, "I'm real sorry to hear about your Grandpa. My Grandma died not long ago an' I know how it hurts." And that's all she said an' then she went away an', you know, I did feel better 'cos I knew she knew - you know, she - knew. I don't know, it made it seem as if it was OK to feel so bad, 'cos in the family, you know, everyone was thinking about Grandma an' how we could help her not be so sad an' it felt a bit like we shouldn't be feeling sad too. So I expect those folk you work with were glad you told them your story about Grandpa 'cos they will know you know what it feels like. It sort of gives you the right to say something.' The spindly legs dangling from the high kitchen stool and the bizarre appearance of this waif caught between adulthood and childhood, were oddly at variance with the maturity of her perception.

'What a wise person you are at times!' Her mother said wonderingly. 'And you're probably right about this. But you know me - ever anxious not to look a fool!'

Their tete-a-tete was broken at that point by the fumbling entrance of a bleary eyed Bob still bearing the marks of a crumpled sheet down the left side of his face.

'Why didn't you wake me, dear?' he asked with a wide yawn.

'Hadn't the heart. You looked so peaceful and Steph was asleep anyway.'

'Wanna tea, Pops?' Vicky was back to her modern teenager guise again.

'Love one, Vicks!' Bob strolled over and picked up the paper from the floor where it had been discarded earlier. He took a seat at the table beside Eileen and recoiled with a start as he went to lay the Daily Mail down.

'What on earth is all - this?' His gesture took in the vast pile of green leaves.

'Don't you recognize leaves when you see them?' Eileen teased.

'But what are they for?'

In a conspiratorial stage whisper Eileen confided, 'These, my dear fellow, are an attempt to hide your youngest son's knees from the combined stare of two hundred pairs of eyes.' Then raising her head proudly and throwing back her shoulders, she proclaimed with a dramatic flourish, 'He has been selected to represent Edgbaston Primary School in their major production destined eventually for Hollywood! He - wait for it! - has been selected out of a cast of thousands to be - ' Eileen paused a long moment for maximum effect. '... a bush!'

Bob's broad smile reached his eyes and Eileen felt a rush of relief. The sleep had done him good and whatever horrors he had had to contend with today he was back on track for the moment.

'Well, he'll probably get even that wrong!' Bob's twinkling eyes took any malice out of his words. Nick's amazing propensity for clumsiness was a family byword.

'Better go and get my work finished,' Vicky declared and disappeared on the word, leaving her parents still smiling and drinking tea.

'She's like mercury that girl - one minute as stubborn and difficult as can be and next all sensitivity and commonsense!' Eileen shook her head at the enigma that was her firstborn. 'Be back in a jiffy but I must just check Tim's in bed.'

He was, but still reading. She understood his reluctance to put the book away. The whole family were avid readers. After ensuring his light was out and would stay so, she tapped on the door of the girls' room. Rachel was head down at her desk and mumbled simply, ' I know, Mum, I'm watching the time. Nearly finished,' pre-empting her mother's warning. There was no sign of Vicky so there might yet be a chance of a quick word with her alone. She was in the sitting room looking up a word in the dictionary.

'Oh there you are! Just wanted to say - thanks for the tea and the chat. You've made me feel better than I've felt all day.' Eileen accompanied her words with a hug deliberately brief so Vicky would no have opportunity to reject her advance and ruin the effect of her earlier comfort. For once Vicky did not seem repulsed by the contact.

'That's OK, Mum, what are daughters for after all!' Her voice mimicked her mother's and they both grinned at each other before Eileen returned to the kitchen.

'You two girls seemed very matey this evening,' Bob remarked once the rhythmic clip, clip, clip of Eileen's scissors had become established.

'Yeeees', she was thinking rapidly as she drew out the word. Should she confide in him about the Flanaghans or had he enough of his own troubles. 'I was telling her about one of our families. They're having to make some difficult decisions. And we're involved too - we're having to think about how we feel about it all.'

'Want to tell me about it or is it too sore?' Bob's outwardly casual enquiry was a veneer. He was unusually sensitive about these things. Probably because of his own experiences, she thought.

'OK. I'll go first and then you can tell me about your day.'

It was good to spill out all her insecurity, all her pain to Bob. There was no need to wrap it up in order to protect her image - he knew her inside out and loved her just the same with all her imperfections.

'Well, for once I think our Vicky has got it right' Bob agreed. 'Don't be so hard on yourself. What happened with your Dad, happened. You were a great daughter. Just because you wouldn't kill him off doesn't mean he died angry with you. He was angry with that horrible disease - and you know as well as I do, when we're angry we usually lash out at those we are closest too - because we know they'll understand and still love us even when we show them our worst side. It was only because your Dad loved you so much that he got so mad with you.'

'Yes, I do know that deep down,' Eileen sighed. 'I also know that I don't think any the worse of folk if they show their emotion so I shouldn't be so annoyed with myself when I do. But we aren't always rational people, are we?'

'Well, you certainly aren't!' His affectionate pat on her arm took any sting out of his words and they both grinned. 'You wouldn't be the girl I married if you suddenly made sense!'

A bantering exchange of incivilities, was interrupted by the appearance of Rachel in a skimpy T-shirt which masqueraded as a nightdress. Her warm embrace for each in turn was reminiscent of her early days when she had been the most demonstrative of all their children.

'Did the physics go all right?' Eileen asked.

'Sort of. Vicky helped me a bit 'cos I hate doing 'electricity' and I can't sort of understand what happens when you stick these different things into circuits. Haven't a clue what a resistor is when it's at home! But she sorted it out - well, I hope she did! I got some answers anyway and that should keep the Old Phantom from stalking me for a day or two.'

She accompanied her reference to the physics teacher with a dramatic expression of a ghost bearing down on them menacingly although the grey T-shirt on her skinny frame presented a figure nearer farce than horror. And her face, now washed clean of the thick white make up had a youthful freshness far from the sinister cadaverous features she was attempting to portray.

'How on earth did Mr Farnham get such a horrible nickname,' Eileen's eyes twinkled.

'Well, apparently, he always used to do this experiment with each new class. He got them all - the whole class - to hold hands round the lab. An' then he sent a current through them all to teach them about conduction. But anyway, one year, the boys, knowing that's what he was going to do, rigged it so the thing short curcuited. The Old Phantom got a shock himself - PsPszzappp - you know, when he went to connect them all up to the current. They said he went white as a sheet - hair on end - shaking. So he looked like a ghost - Phantom, see?' They all laughed at the story.

'No respect for their elders these days,' Bob threw up his hands in mock horror.

'That's right, Dad! Gone to the dogs the modern generation!' And with that Rachel skipped merrily out of reach and out of the room to bed.

A lumping noise on the stairs indicated Vicky's descent a few minutes later. More decorously attired with a thick navy dressing gown she too had shed years with the removal of her make up and the brushing of her dark hair. Her goodnight was briefer and no physical contact was made. Instead she placed both hands around the doorframe, swung the upper part of her body round the corner and called breezily, 'Night, Momsy! Night, Popsy!'

'Night, Vicks Vapour Rub,' her parents chorused with a ritual that spanned 12 years.

'I'm glad you're my parents!'

She vanished without waiting for a response, suddenly made shy by this expression of appreciation.

Her parents shared this rare moment with a deep sense of contentment. Another cup of tea seemed an appropriate response. It was only once they were settled back again into their seats, Eileen busy with her leaves and Bob spreading the paper wide, that Eileen ventured another enquiry about his day. She saw his eyes darken and the muscles of his face tighten. She reached across and covered his hand with hers.

'Only if you want to.' Her voice was gentle.

He twisted his fingers through hers watching the changing pattern of their intertwining but seeing instead the mangled bodies of those teenage boys. They had been driving far too fast along an open country road. The driver was a lad who had only passed his test a couple of months earlier, and that car - his father's - was far too powerful for a youngster exhilarated by a new sense of power and freedom.

'An articulated lorry was coming the other way. The guy - the driver - he said they seemed to swerve - avoiding a a rabbit or something. The car just skidded right out of control - ploughed straight into him. What a nightmare! The guy was a wreck! Not his fault! But imagine watching them coming for you - nothing you could do to stop them!' Bob shuddered violently, his face contorted with horror. 'He slammed on his brakes but - wouldn't have made much difference - you know, 'cos of the speed of the other car. I tried to get him to move away - you know - not look too closely. But - no - it was like he was sort of transfixed. At one point he went to the edge of the road - vomited his heart up. But even after - he just couldn't seem to look away. And of course, we had our job to do - so I couldn't really stay with him. The driver and the front passenger - they were killed outright, the medics said. Lads of 17, Eils! Just the age of our Vicky! The lad in the back - still breathing, you know, when we all arrived. We cut him out - the car was just a tangled mess - he was carted off to St Joseph's. In such a mess. Such a mess. Doesn't look hopeful for him either. Good grief, Eils, if he was mine I wouldn't - I really wouldn't - want him to survive that. Never be any good. But what a waste.' Bob's tortured look was reflected in Eileen's eyes. 'Three kids just wiped out. Three families destroyed.'

'Doesn't bear thinking about!' Eileen's voice was a bare murmur.

'I never get used to these ones with youngsters involved. Must be too soft. But, you know, Eils, sometimes I can actually see Tim or Vicks or one of them lying there. It's such a nightmare, I sort of freeze. Of course, you have to stop thinking and get on with the job but it's damned difficult sometimes - not to just sit down and cry from the sheer waste of it all.'

Releasing her hand he thumped the table so hard vinyl leaves cascaded on to the floor. He buried his head in his hands with a groan that tore at her heart. She rose and wrapped him against her body rocking him as she would a distressed child, smoothing the thinning grey hair with her hand. He clung to her fiercely, desperately trying to eradicate those nightmarish scenes. After a time he lifted tortured eyes and asked pleadingly, 'Eils, what would we do - if it was one of ours? You know - when that lad was carted off today, more dead than alive - d'you know what I was wondering?'

She shook her head.

'I was wondering - wondering if his parents would let them have his heart and eyes and everything. What a thought, eh?! Not even really dead yet - thinking about chopping him up for spare parts. I sometimes wonder -

would I have the courage - when it came to the crunch, you know. OK, I agree in principle, as you know, but it freaks me out to think of anyone carving any of my own kids up.' A fierce tightening of his arms as he contemplated this new horror, almost sent her off balance.

Steadying herself she soothed, 'Don't torture yourself, Bob, with what might be. It hasn't happened to us, so far, thank God - probably never will. If it does, well, I think people get the strength when they need it. I believe that - really I do.' With the last words she took his face in her hands and looked deep into his eyes. 'I feel for you - feeling all this tragedy so much. But I'm glad you're like you are. It must be horrendous to be brutalised by it - you know. Or desensitised so you just don't feel it any more.'

A long silent holding of each other close conveyed a mutual sympathy of feeling broken only by the sound of the clock and kettle.

'What a couple of old weepies we are today. Must be getting too old for all this caper.' Her words were deliberately light. No point in encouraging bad dreams or raging insomnia. 'There's a film on tonight I'd like to see - need some powerful distraction. Watch it with me with the horlicks and the warmed slippers and the pipe, Grandad?'

'Sure thing, Grandma. Bags me to make the drinks, though - I can't abide the weak rubbish you call Horlicks.'

The film was, after all, only mediocre but it served the purpose. A sound night's sleep was too much for either to expect but their trauma was eased by the sharing as well as by the constant trivialities of normal family life.

CHAPTER 4

The Consultant's Daughter

As Roger left the Unit after that Monday meeting to discuss Peter Flanaghan's fate, he was preoccupied with thoughts of the various members of the staff who had contributed to the discussion today. How little he really knew of them. Oh, he knew the ones who were efficient and calm in a crisis. He knew the ones who sought confirmation for what they had to do; the ones who questioned orders; the ones who gave that extra something to their caring. But outside of the Unit he knew pretty much nothing of how they lived their lives. Yet it was largely those other experiences that made them react to situations like that of the Flanaghan family in such different ways.

Wendy, the new girl - she clearly had strong views about life. There were Catholics and Catholics, but she was obviously one of the ones who took her religious beliefs seriously. The clash between her views and the student's passionate opinions had shown she could remain calm under fire but she was definitely not going to be pushed into something she didn't approve of. Seemed like a pleasant, gentle soul and she obviously won the confidence of the parents. But sometimes it was the quiet ones, the ones who didn't feel empowered to come out with their opinions, who couldn't cope with the outcome. A burning need to right a wrong or just to unburden themselves of the weight of the knowledge of what had been done, compelled them to go off and tell somebody. And the Pro-lifers were good listeners. So were the press! Yes, he'd better make an effort to chat to Wendy.

Roger didn't know what to make of Jo Manson's outburst. To begin with she was just passing through the Unit, not a permanent member of the team. You couldn't get to know all these temporary faces and how they ticked. And the situation became more tricky when people introduced their own personal experience to set a precedent for all cases. He knew, probably better than most, how dominating such catastrophic experiences could be. But there were ways of using them which were persuasive and there were ways which simply irritated other people. Maybe it was Catherine Woollard's job to try to keep tabs on her fluctuating band of nurses. Might be useful to discuss that with her.

Eileen Shorten, now, she had introduced her experience with her father in an altogether more mature way. She wasn't bombastic - wasn't demanding attention - wasn't setting her family up as the definitive answer to this thorny problem. Or was it rather that her quiet rather sad reflective comments didn't make your hackles rise like the hectoring tones Jo had adopted? If he was honest he felt a bit resentful at the student's attitude simply because she was a student. He could respect the vast amount of experience Eileen had under her belt and somehow that gave her a greater right to speak out. But of course, that wasn't entirely fair. Jo had had powerful experiences too. She had years of experience in another discipline too. In any case, her student status didn't make her any less a person with opinions. Nowadays the students were taught to be more assertive, more challenging of received wisdom. She was probably just a product of the system. But he knew he himself instinctively gravitated to the quiet, gentle ones. Equally a product of his upbringing and education! Brave girl, Eileen to expose herself like that - he admired her courage. Ring of truth there you didn't often hear.

Tom - yes, he must find out what was eating Tom. Far too many occasions where his brusqueness upset the team. Tensions were high enough in the nursery without conflict among the team members. Almost on a impulse he decided to seek the registrar out now while it was fresh in his mind.

Roger judged that Tom would probably be in the lab at this hour of the day so he deliberately set his path in that direction. The familiar precisely combed head of thick auburn hair was visible at the end of the corridor as he turned the corner and he metaphorically crossed his fingers for courage. The love of Tom's professional life was the work he did in the lab. If anyone took an interest in it his evident enthusiasm transformed him from the rather boorish doctor into a passionate, crusading scientist.

'How goes it, Tom?' Roger asked, peering in at the scrabbling white mice Tom was examining.

'Well. Very well,' Tom replied, still intent on his scrutiny. 'Last phase starts tomorrow and if the the next batch react the same as this lot we should be home and dry.'

'Is this the ovarian transplant study, still?'

'It is indeed! This is my Achilles heel - if the whistle blowers want to get me! But I don't confess all - not like in the Nursery. What they don't know about they can't blab about.'

'Very different situation', Roger spoke quietly. 'They don't need to be involved here - you only need to be assured of the integrity of your lab staff. In the nursery they are all involved.'

'Maybe, but I still think - they won't have to take the rap if the case goes to court.'

'D'you think I should just do my own thing and not consult them, then?'

'Well, if it were me I'd rather just discuss it with the parents and a medical colleague and then do whatever we agree is best.'

'Doesn't the nursing input count for anything?'

'They aren't responsible for the decisions. They should just do what we decide the baby needs.'

'Doesn't that make them into automatons - technicians?'

Tom shrugged but said nothing more.

'I actually came across to ask if you were doing anything tomorrow evening,' Roger changed the subject suddenly.

Thinking he was about to be asked to take an extra night on call, Tom instantly replied that he had nothing arranged.

'Good, then how about coming to dinner tomorrow night? My wife, Virginia's a superb cook and I'd like to get to know you a bit better. I realized with a bit of a shock today at that meeting that I don't know much about any of the team outside of work. Not that I intend to throw a series of dinner parties!' he added laughingly.

Tom was startled. His relationship with Roger had never strayed outside the professional. But a good meal in convivial company might be just the tonic he needed.

'Bring a partner if you like. I don't know if there is anyone?' Roger's tone was deliberately matter of fact. He had no intention of prying. He knew Tom's marriage had foundered just before he came to work at Alexandra's. It had been blurted out one day when an innocent enquiry had touched a raw nerve and Roger had avoided any reference to wives or children since.

'No. No-one.' The curt response closed the subject.

Roger's instructions on how to reach his home were easy to follow. But Tom was unprepared for the grandeur of the establishment. The carefully manicured lawns and flamboyant flower beds formed a perfect foil for the magnificent architecture of the house itself. With steeply-pitched roofs, and turrets at either end, the grey stone was complemented and softened by the tumbling riot of palest pink roses on either side of the great oak door. At the sound of his wheels crunching on the gravel the door swung open and Roger appeared as if he had had nothing better to do than await the arrival of his guest.

Tom instantly wished he had brought something more sophisticated than the bottle of Safeway's wine. Inside did nothing to make him more comfortable. Everything breathed taste and elegance. He would have given a lot to have a grubby dog rush out of nowhere and dishevel the exact symmetry of the cushions on the settee. Even a fellow guest being the first to spoil the beautiful folds of the crisp creation which was in another life a navy blue serviette, would have reassured him that he might breath normally. But there was no-one else out of step in this perfection but himself.

Roger, apparently oblivious to his acute discomfort, led him to a seat in the window where they could survey the brilliance of the garden. Holding his Martini in a grip more suited to a baseball bat than a fine Waterford Crystal glass, Tom enquired who was the mastermind behind the landscaping.

'Ginny. She's the artistic one - knows about colours and shapes and textures and what will look right where. I leave it all to her. The garden and the house. She decides all that. She's an interior designer.'

The pride in Roger's voice was unmistakable. 'I can't tell my ambers from my bronzes!'

'Nonsense! You are my chief critic.' The low contralto voice held a hint of laughter. Tom rose to his feet as Virginia entered the room. Tall, ash blond, she looked more like a magazine illustration than a part of life. She advanced with outstretched hand. Tom's closer gaze took in the slightly irregular white teeth, the rather angular contours and the slow blink of eyes not quite adapted to her contact lenses. No, it wasn't that she was a beauty in the conventional sense. But she had this air of serenity that was more attractive than a superficial prettiness.

'My wife, Virginia.' Again that ring of pride in Roger's voice.

Her hand grasped Tom's warmly as she smiled her welcome.

'Don't take any notice of Roger's modesty. He is a dab hand with the paintbrush and the hoe!' Her affection was evident as she took the proffered glass from her husband and sank down into a chair beside her guest.

'Are you interested in gardening, Tom? May I call you, Tom?' she enquired.

'Yes, of course. Please do. Well, I wouldn't say, interested exactly. I do have a garden and I cut the grass and weed and stick plants in, but it's more a job that has to be done than a real interest.'

'So, what are your hobbies?'

'Well, I sail a bit and I love hill walking.' The usually reticent Tom was drawn into a detailed and vivid description of his recent escapades by the genuine warmth of her questioning. It was only when she rose to attend to something in the kitchen that he realized he had been doing almost all the talking. What an intent listener she was!

Whatever her task, it was soon completed and she reappeared to inform them that the meal was ready. By now the splendour of the table and the exquisite blend of flavours came as no surprise to Tom. But his panic had, by this time, deserted him in the face of the relaxed ease of his hosts. For this brief interlude he was as much a part of all this grandeur as they were. They made it so.

As naturally as she had asked about his sailing and his home, Virginia enquired about his family.

'Divorced.' Tom felt again the pain of the admission. It had been a woundingly acrimonious affair, the separation and finally the divorce. He'd have found it easier if the contention had been about money or even if she'd had an affair. But it hadn't been that way. Angela had been desperate to start a family once they'd bought the house and got 'the essentials'. Funny how 'wants' became 'essentials' once you had the bare minimum in place. He'd wanted to wait until they were better placed financially but she was single minded about the babies. She wanted four, no point in delaying starting. She wanted to be young enough to be their friend as well as their mother. Loving her, wanting her to be satisfied with her life as his wife, he had succumbed to her emotional pressure.

But it hadn't worked out that way. She just didn't get pregnant to order. After two increasingly tearful years she took herself off to the doctor, who referred her to the specialists. Her passionate desire for motherhood propelled her through all those ignominious infertility tests. From the outset, Tom had steadfastly resisted any efforts to get him to go along too. Oh, yes, he'd ferry her about so she could be poked and invaded as much as she chose to be. But no, he wouldn't have any tests done himself. No need. He knew there was nothing wrong with him. He performed all right, didn't he?

But in the end their family doctor had rung him and asked him to go to the surgery to discuss Angela's problem. Grumbling, he had nevertheless gone as requested.

It had shocked him to the core to hear that Angela was seriously depressed. How could he have been so blind to her symptoms? Fine sort of a doctor he must be. But cobblers' children were the ones with holes in their shoes. Was it his fault? Should he take her on holiday, buy her a bit of jewellery? What should he do?

'It's not a holiday she wants, Tom, it's a baby.'

'Well, I can't just produce one of those! I can't help it if she's infertile.'

'But she isn't, Tom. She's had all the tests needed and there doesn't appear to be anything at all wrong with her. Tubes are patent, ovulation normal. All working fine.'

'So, what are you saying?'

'It takes two to tango, Tom,' Alan Bryant's voice was gentle. 'What I'm saying is - if we are to move forward I really think you should go for a test.'

He saw from Tom's dilating pupils how abhorrent the idea was to him.

'I know it's a horrid prospect and we all like to keep our private lives private - especially us doctors! We're not good at seeing ourselves as members of the human race - not when it comes to our own health. But I am seriously worried about Angela. I know it has cost her dearly to have all these tests herself. She feels violated in many ways. But she went through it and I suspect she tried to keep a brave face for you. I do think you owe it to her to at least go and give a specimen, old chap. It won't be nearly as much of an invasion of privacy as what she's been through. And once we know you're OK, we can start thinking of the options. No adoption agency will look at her case without your test results.'

Adoption! Tom recoiled in amazement. It had come to that! He had hardly begun to get seriously anxious about the delay in conceiving. Suited his books very nicely to have a bit longer to amass the wherewithal to bring up and educate his children.

In the face of all the circumstances he couldn't refuse. He had gone along to the clinic and produced a specimen to order. For a reason he couldn't articulate he didn't want Angela to accompany him - not then - not when he went for the follow up appointment. There were certain things a chap had to just grit his teeth about and get on with. If it helped her to contemplate adoption that might make her relax and not be so intense about conceiving. That was sometimes all it took to make a woman pregnant.

'I'm sorry, Tom, but both numbers and motility are greatly reduced.' Tom stared at the sympathetic grey eyes as the message penetrated his stupefied brain.

'There's been some mistake ...' his voice sounded as strangled as his emotions.

'No mistake. You are almost entirely infertile.'

It couldn't be so. He came from a long line of virile men. The family was positively hotching with children.

The next 20 minutes passed in a daze for Tom. He couldn't tell Angela. He'd have to. Did he want this infertility specialist to tell her instead? Or their GP? She knew he was getting the result today. There was no escaping telling her. What about treatment - could the count be improved? How could he face the endless examination of those parts of his very being which were most private?

When he eventually escaped those sterile magnolia clinic walls, he was shivering in spite of the balmy spring morning. How could the birds chirrup so merrily! How could those women on the park bench giggle at their own silly jokes, as they rocked prams and chattered together - idly chattering - so blase about the bundles of life they bounced. The hugely pregnant girl he passed seemed to mock his impotence.

Unable to face going home to the blue questioning eyes Angela would raise as he entered, he dived into the first restaurant he came to, slunk into the darkest corner and huddled into a pretence of reading the menu.

'What would you like, sir?' The waitress stood, pencil poised.

Two hundred million sperm! That's what he wanted!

'A black coffee, please.' It sounded a pathetic substitute.

'Anything with it, sir?' He shook his head willing her to leave him alone in his misery.

The telling had been every bit as bad as he had anticipated. Angela had actually shrunk away from him as he tried to explain.

'You - you wasted all these months! If you had gone - gone when I first said about it, I wouldn't have had to have all those examinations; all those tests; the anaesthetic ...' Dawning realization even as she spoke turned any hope of sympathy for his plight into ashes. 'There was nothing wrong with me. It was you all the time!' The venom grew more bitter and he would never forget the cruel words she'd flung at him from the heat of her anger and the bitterness that came with the death of any hope she had clung to.

He had half believed that the rejection of the closed bedroom door that night would turn out to be a passing fury. Then they could talk this thing out and decide what was best to do. OK, he'd get used to adoption in time if that's what she wanted. But the closed door became a routine and then a cold certainty. She would not forget. Would not forgive. There was no talking, no understanding, no consideration of the options.

In the end the separation had been an inevitable development. It had actually been easier to move into another flat than to endure the farce their being together had become. Now he did not listen for the door opening and wait for her to sneak up behind him and slip her arms around his neck as she nuzzled into his auburn curls. With no-one there to open a door he had no vain expectations. Increasingly he threw himself into work. His bitterness turned into scorn for womankind who could at a moment's notice turn from sweetly sensuous into frigid monuments of disdain.

Something of his pain came through in his tight lipped 'Divorced'. Virginia inclined slightly towards him as she murmured, 'I'm sorry. That must be hard. Any children?' His every instinct was to tell this gracious impeccably groomed woman to shut up and mind her own business but he was not so lost to propriety and simply uttered a bald, 'No'.

Both hosts were startled by the expression in his eyes. Before they had a chance to steer the conversation into safer waters, he abruptly turned to Virginia and asked, 'Have you?' He was too caught up in his own raw emotion to notice the change which came over her face. It was after all scarcely perceptible.

Her answer was a simple, 'Two. One of each.'

'Very organized. How old?'

'Our daughter, Eleanor, she's 23. Damian, he's 21.'

'And what are they doing - away at University acquiring three or four degrees like their father?' Tom tried so hard to inject a lighter note into the conversation, to project his thoughts on to this normal happy family.

'Damian is - away at University, anyway. Studying law actually - doesn't take after his father there - never any interest in biology or bodies.' She grimaced to indicate his dislike of medical matters. 'Eleanor, she's just at home.'

There was a curious stillness in the air as she spoke. Tom couldn't place what had changed as they outwardly continued to ply their forks and swallow chicken marengo.

'I'm sorry not to meet her.' She must be quite a girl if she combined her father's brilliant mind and her mother's taste and elegance. Perhaps she was a rebel. Refusing to conform to what was expected of a child of such a family.

'You can meet her later, if you wish.' Roger's words were even and curiously without expression.

'Out dazzling the neighbourhood, is she?'

'No, she's just upstairs. She isn't able to go out.'

Tom wondered idly why she wasn't eating with them and concluded that her father's work colleagues would make dull company for a vibrant young woman in her early 20s. There was no sound of other life in the house but it was so vast that was hardly surprising.

His compliments to Virginia on her almond gateau were genuine. She seemed to excel at everything. Best meal he'd had in ages. Fortunate fellow, Roger. Modestly disclaiming any extraordinary skill, Virginia asked him about his own taste in food and they were soon exchanging reminiscences about Italian and Chinese fare in the way of old friends. Roger emerged as a connoisseur of port and the two men rootled through Roger's not inconsiderable cellar for a time, oblivious to the weighty problems which normally threw them together in serious discussion.

It was after ten when Tom finally declined any more coffee and muttered that he really ought to be making a move.

'I'll take you up and introduce you to Eleanor,' Roger answered, rising and relieving him of his empty cup. 'Perhaps I should warn you - you might find it difficult to meet her. She's not like other girls.' So she probably was rebellious. Tom wondered if she'd be rude to him, just ignore him perhaps. Sounded as if she was quite an embarrassment. He felt a sudden pang of compassion for Roger having to apologise for his only daughter like that. All was not quite perfect in this seemingly flawless household. Perversely that made him feel more comfortable.

Leading the way, Roger took Tom up the curved ornate staircase. Magnificent portraits hung at intervals and Tom had a sense of unreality as he scanned this other world so at variance with his simple surburban conformity. These two oozed a sort of breeding he could only dimly comprehend. It made him uneasy suddenly that he might well be betraying his own humble origins. He was a man more used to cheap prints than original paintings; to durable pottery than to fine porcelain. Not that they had been in the least standoffish or superior. But that's what somebody once said, wasn't it? 'Those who care where they sit don't matter, and those who matter don't care where they sit!' True here. But every facet of the Carshalton's lives - their way of speaking, their acceptance of such a standard of living, betrayed their backgrounds and their status. They didn't need to tell anyone they were in a higher league.

The corridor on the second floor was furnished more simply - colours brighter - strangely incongruous in this house of muted tones. At one end two rag dolls side by side lolled drunkenly on a wooden chest, gingham frocks and broiderie anglais aprons cheekily rustic amid the elegance. Relics of Eleanor's youth he supposed. Tom guessed this corridor had once housed the army of servants needed to run such a vast Victorian household. What did the Carshaltons do with so much room? Probably entertained lavishly. Or perhaps their only daughter had taken over this upper story as her own flat. It must be about as big as his entire house. Even these upper regions were palatial by his standards. But they must have a fair income, this successful professional couple and what else to lavish it all on than home and family.

The room at the end of the corridor they entered was surprisingly dimly lit. Tom supposed no 23-year-old would be in bed at this early hour, so what was she doing in so little light? As his eyes adjusted, he made out the outline of a single bed with a flounced cover loosely scattered over its uneven shape. Movement made the light dance on the huge brass bedhead and the rails down each side. Taking in the spacious ceilings and the orderly neatness of a room almost too tidy for human habitation he noted the irregularity of the coverlet was the only thing in the room to disturb its uncanny precision. It was as if it was a monument to a departed child. You heard of families who preserved rooms as shrines to dead children. His mind did a double take. Rails down each side? His eyes flew back to the bed.

By now Roger had switched on a side lamp and a gentle glow pervaded the sheltering gloom. Still in silence he moved towards the bed and turning the cover with a careful hand, he revealed a form which made Tom, with all his years in paediatrics, recoil in sick horror. Perhaps it was experience, perhaps it was a knowledge of his colleague, that made Roger keep his eyes turned from Tom's face at first. His whole attention was devoted to the creature in the bed as he gently caressed her shoulder and stooped to kiss the lank dark hair matted from the constant movement from side to side. Eleanor's features were a cruel caricature. Her mouth drooled, the tongue inpervious to the stream of saliva soaking her pillow. The eyes in another being could have been lustrous; instead they stared uncomprehendingly from sunken sockets, the shaggy brows gathered in an ugly frown. Spastic hands bent at an incongruous angle grasped and ungrasped the air as if constantly seeking the reassurance of solid boundaries. Beneath the cover, the contorted legs made a bizarre outline. The unmistakable smell of incontinence completed the picture which appalled Tom's every sense.

It was a long moment before Roger said in a voice Tom hardly recognized, 'Tom, meet my only daughter, Eleanor. Eleanor, this is my colleague, Dr Tom Faithful, from the hospital.' For one spellbound moment Tom suspected Roger of sarcastic mimicry. But one startled look at the father's face and he recognized the gesture for what it really was. An innate courtesy made him treat even this travesty of a daughter with the chivalry he accorded to everyone.

Tom's own breeding was not the product of generations of nannies. He felt an awkwardness and embarrassment that froze his lips as he mumbled, 'Hello, Eleanor.'

'Tom is here for a meal with us, Eleanor. We work together but we don't have much time to get to know one another so we thought an evening at home might fit the bill.' It was unnerving. Talking so politely to such a non-person. 'He asked about you, so I wanted to introduce you. Hope I haven't disturbed your sleep. We'll leave you to rest now, darling, but I'll ask Annie to come in and make you comfortable first.'

Excusing himself for a moment Roger left through a door opening to one side of the large window and Tom heard a murmur of voices before he reappeared with a trim middle-aged woman in a blue overall who nodded a greeting to him before gathering together the essentials for a change of bedding for her charge.

'We'll leave the women to it, Tom. And I'll show you my latest hobby. I've decided the garden needs a pond and I'm trying my hand at stonemasonry - not very well!' How could he sound so matter of fact and behave so normally?

Tom scarcely heard the gentle flow of Roger's outlining of his plans and the obstacles he'd encountered in the pursuit of his latest enterprise. Moving through a different part of the building - noting the passing loveliness of an antique escritoire, the defracted light of a thousand crystal droplets of the hall chandelier - he was all the time grappling with the ghastly incongruity between this gracious beauty and the stark ugliness he had just witnessed. How could these parents, so attuned to the refinements of a life he could only dimly appreciate, cope with such a catastrophic violation of perfection?

He felt he should say something. What was there to say? A hundred encounters with the parents of all the children he had ever cared for did not prepare him for this moment.

The cool refreshing of the evening breeze restored a measure of composure to his turbulent thoughts. Striding across the great striped lawn in the friendly half light, Tom at last found courage to speak.

'Was it brain damage - Eleanor, I mean?' His question sounded crass. He hadn't meant it to be so. A small sigh preceded Roger's calm response.

'Yes, Ginny had a long and very difficult birth. We were in Czechoslovakia at the time. I'd gone for a week-long conference. Ginny came along for a break. She was 36 weeks. We thought it would be nice - going together - have a few days holiday there before we returned. Last chance before Ginny had the children and couldn't just up sticks and accompany me so easily.'

They arrived at the pond and Roger gestured extravagantly at the piles of carefully sculpted stone still looking for those cementing plants and friendly mosses which would transform it from a stark wall into a coherent entity. The water sparkled in the half light and both men were grateful for the diversion and the comfort of the evening gloom. A statue of a heron stood abandoned to one side and a trough half filled with water provided a temporary habitat for the plants which would soften the contours and nourish the wildlife when Roger's vision was realized. They talked cursorily of the plans for this latest development in the Carshalton's garden, neither really caring at that moment what became of the vision.

It was Roger who returned to the subject of Eleanor, even as he inched one of the stones into an angle nearer to the water. He was hundreds of miles away and deep inside a nightmare.

'Ginny started in labour during the night - the very day after we arrived there. We rushed her off to the hospital but they're in a time warp out there. Well, they certainly were 23 years ago. The whole experience was a nightmare. I begged them to Section her but there was a double problem. The language barrier we could overcome because there were other medics at the conference who could interpret for us. The real problem was that they were adamant their style of management was every bit as good as ours. In the end Eleanor was born - no, dragged out with Kiellands - after a three-hour second stage, moribund. Ginny had to have a GA to remove a retained placenta - they whisked her off to some room - said I couldn't accompany her. So I stayed with the baby - sure she was just going to die - she looked so ghastly. The paediatrician, he was so unhurried it was unreal - like one of those movies you see in slow motion. I'd already antagonised them by offering suggestions about Ginny's management - they were in no mood to brook interference with the baby. Well, let's just say they did everything they thought fit but - it wasn't what we would do here. The damage was already done anyway. The first few weeks just added problems on to an already bleak prospect. They kept Eleanor alive - at four weeks we flew her back to this country. It took us a while - a while to realize the full extent of the damage. But basically - she's never been able to do anything for herself.'

'I just don't know what to say,' Tom blurted out his inadequacy. 'I'm so desperately sorry.'

'Thanks. I know. It comes as a shock to other people. But Ginny and I - well, we've got used to it and, of course, she's our daughter so we love her and that makes it easier.'

'Does it?' Tom marvelled at his philosophy. 'Doesn't it make it all the harder to see your precious child so ... so ... damaged?'

'Well, of course, we wish she was normal and could respond to us and so on, but we know she can't. Loving her - just loving her - that helps us to see beyond the contortions and the incontinence and the grunting and the dependence and recognize the being trapped in this shell.'

'Your wife, Virginia, she seems so - I don't know - so serene.'

'Yes, that describes Ginny exactly. She's a pretty remarkable girl, is Ginny. She has this belief, you see. She believes that parents like us have been singled out by God to look after these special creatures. I'm afraid I can't subscribe to that kind of thing - seems like a cruel God who'd do this kind of thing deliberately.' Roger shuddered slightly at the thought - or was it the cool night air? Tom couldn't know.

'But when you live with someone who believes that so completely - just takes the whole thing so calmly - well, it affects you after a while. My anger and frustration at what had happened seemed disloyal to Ginny - and in a way a rejection of Eleanor after a while. I wish I could share Ginny's feelings about it all. I'm too much of a scientist and not enough of a believer to ever really see it that way. But I know it's a whole lot less difficult to deal with if you stop ranting and raving and accept it - whatever interpretation you put on it. It took me many years to get to this point though.'

'Having Damian - that helped. Well, in some ways. It's helped me, anyway. He is just so normal. But it hurts Ginny I know - probably more than me - to compare the two children. Everything falls into Damian's lap, somehow. He's bright, outgoing, lots of friends, doing well at University. It helps me to hear about his progress. And he's a keen sporstman - fencing, rowing. Much more able in that direction than I ever was. But Ginny - well, of course she's pleased when Damian does well, but she grieves too - grieves for what Eleanor has missed.'

'And you never mention this when we have discussions in the Unit,' Tom was awed. 'Isn't it too much to hear the opinions of the others knowing what you know - first hand so to speak?'

'I don't bring it up for several reasons, not all of them very creditable.' Roger's smile was wry. 'For one thing it took me years to get to my present position in relation to my own daughter. And who's to say that position won't change again at some point. And then I feel it would stifle others. You can't argue with personal experience and it won't ever be everyone's experience - mercifully! So I feel it would give me an unfair amount of clout. Especially as I'm the boss. It's hard enough for some of the team to state their opinion without me adding that dimension.'

What a thoroughly honourable man Roger Carshalton was, Tom mused. He doubted he would see it like that. He had already let a much less traumatic experience sour his relations with his colleagues.

'And then our way of dealing with the situation - it wouldn't be right for everyone else. Without Ginny - her uncomplaining acceptance of the whole thing - I'm not sure I could have coped. You'd have to go long way to find another Ginny.' Roger's voice lingered over her name.

'If they'd asked me then, 23 years ago what I'd prefer - Eleanor as she is, or to allow her to die - I'm pretty sure I'd have chosen the latter. But they never did ask us. If I feel so ambivalent about it, what right have I to inflict such a burden on others? But if I said that, that would inhibit other people too - stop them stating their beliefs.

'And there's another reason for not speaking about it. I very much value my privacy. I just don't want other people's pity or sympathy or whatever. My private life is separate from my professional life. And, I don't know, but I suspect - and here's the discreditable bit - I suspect that I don't want to ... to tarnish my image at work. What a low thought. There is still a sort of stigma attached to handicap. And when it's severe and totally incapacitating like Eleanor's it does foster attitudes and barriers and so on. I'm not proud of my periods where I wish she would just slip away from some chest infection. But I do have them - and I have all the advantages of a live-in nurse to care for her. I do spend time with her - pretty much every day - but I rarely ever have to change her or feed her. I simply cannot imagine coming home from a hard day's work and having to do everything for her and get up umpteen times a night to clean her up. But that's what so many families have to do for the rest of the child's life. And Damian - he's well-adjusted - isn't really affected by his sister's disability really. He can live his own life - not like some sibs. So how could I use my experience as an example? It's not by any means typical.'

'I can see what you mean but I must say, your attitude to all of this - well, it's - I don't know - impressive. It must be tempting - to put your point of view, I mean, when people are - you know, dogmatic - about all life being sacred, or parents shouldn't be allowed to choose.'

'Not as tempting as you might think, actually. In a strange kind of way I have a strong desire to protect Eleanor. And not allowing others to use her as an example, to debate the value of her life - it's a form of protection. It sounds convoluted thinking - even to me - but I think - well, parental feelings are not always rational. I must say, I found it incredibly difficult to hear some of my own family trying to disclaim any possible connection with abnormality. You know, the 'nothing like that in our family' syndrome! Well, we had that too!

'What is harder to bear is comparing her lot with that of her peers. I feel a great sadness when I hear other fathers discussing their daughters' successes, their boyfriends, competing for jobs, doing well. It's not just because I can't share in their pride; it's because my daughter has been denied so many of life's rich experiences. She will never be a graduate, a bride, a mother. Life has been cruel to her.' His voice had dropped to a scarcely audible level.

'You make me feel very ashamed.' Tom was astonished at his own words.

'Oh, don't be. I'm no paragon. It's just my circumstances are easier than lots of people's.'

'Did you ask me to dinner to give me a jolt?'

Roger's uncomprehending look was genuine.

'I'm afraid I don't understand what you're getting at. I asked you to dinner - to get to know you better - how you tick. Well, if I'm perfectly honest, I have to confess - I've been a bit worried about how you treat the other staff at times. I vaguely thought - if I understood why you get irritated with them I might be able to smooth things along a little better.'

'I realize I do get ratty with them. I know. I have difficulty trusting them. I could cut my tongue out sometimes. I didn't used to have this problem - not before Angela left me. But I didn't know it was quite so obvious.'

In the confidence of this quiet spot and moved by the insight he had just had into Roger's greater sadness and greater compassion, Tom for the first time felt he could confide in someone. His tale was told haltingly as he felt again the pain of the whole sorry business. Both men had dropped down on to a flat stone beside the pond and Roger idly trailed one finger in the water watching the ripples flow and merge endlessly. Tom sat rigidly, reliving his experience without direct scrutiny.

'So, you see,' Tom concluded, 'I know what you mean - about how it feels - hearing other parents proudly sharing children's progress. My reason's are different - but it hurts just the same. But I've let this hurt affect my relationship with colleagues - yes, especially the females. I'm enormously impressed by the way you've turned a greater hurt into positive good. Everyone is impressed - by your compassion and understanding and courtesy towards everybody and that's without knowing - well, I presume they don't know the full story?' He wasn't sure if anyone at work did know about Eleanor, but the enquiry invoked a quick shake of Roger's head. 'That is humbling.'

'Thank you - you're very kind, Tom. I'm glad we've had this chat. Sometimes we all need to let the tension go in a safe place. I really am so sorry you have such a cross to bear. I shall, of course, respect your confidences absolutely.'

For a long moment they sat silently, each sharing the other's pain. Tom remembered all his envy of Roger - beautiful home, impeccable origins, an elegant and loving wife. Then the stark contrast - that glimpse of Eleanor in all her flexed inaccessibility. He felt sick. Sick because of the cruelty of it all. Sick that he had envied Roger - wanted things to be not so perfect.

The striking of the village clock brought them back to the present and they rose as Tom said, 'I really must be going. I'm afraid I have long outstayed my welcome.'

'Not at all. Glad to have a chat.'

As they approached the house the soft tones of the piano rippled out across the still air. Tom glanced enquiringly at his companion.

'Another of Ginny's accomplishments.'

She was clearly absorbed in her playing and did not notice their return. They both stood watching the fair head, eyes closed revelling in the beauty of the music. It was only when they applauded spontaneously that she startled and reentered their world.

Tom's grasp of her hand was warm as he tried to convey his thanks.

'This has been an incredible evening for me. I shall not forget that amazing chervil and mushroom soup! But most of all I shall not forget Eleanor.'

Her luminous eyes looked into his for a long moment as she retained his hand. 'You must come again - and meet Damian.'

'I'd like that. He sounds to be a son you can be very proud of.'

'We're prejudiced, of course.'

The hall light threw a halo round her blond hair as she stood close to Roger in the doorway to wave a farewell as Tom left.

Letting himself into his silent home, cramped, untidy and tastelessly furnished, his envy had given way to an enormous respect. Sleep was a long time coming, but the self analysis had been healing and he would feel it's refreshing in spite of the physical fatigue of the following morning.

CHAPTER 5

Jo's Conflict

While Tom was being entertained in the elegance of the Carshalton's home, Jo Manson was entering a very different world where her sister, Val, lived. A far greater distance than the 39 miles separated these two residences.

The country bus ground slowly up the hills and Jo, tired from a long shift in the Neonatal Unit, nodded off into an uneasy sleep. They had been more than usually busy with three staff off with the flu, and four new admissions that morning. As she had checked and double checked each activity she carried out, Jo had been anxiously questioning the staff nurse, Karen Tomlinson, working alongside her. Was this the right amount of pressure to exert on the chest wall? Were these electrodes correctly positioned? Was this the correct speed for the formula feed to be injected down the nasogastric tube? Should the stool really be this greenish yellow? She felt hopelessly out of her depth. Her colleague must feel so frustrated and irritated by the endless questions about such routine tasks, when she was so hard pressed herself. But looking after these infants was a very different thing from being in charge of 36 adult surgical patients. There must be such a small margin for error. She was desperately afraid of making a mistake. But then she knew how dearly one paid for a mistake in nursing.

Jo's nursing career had been so much more than a job. Nursing was her life. As a ward sister, she had been dimly aware that her junior staff resented her arriving early and working long beyond the end of her shift. It wasn't really that she didn't trust them but she couldn't expect anyone else to take quite the pride in perfection that she took. Oh, she was renowned for her fairness in making up overtime to her staff. If they stayed on in a crisis, they would be let off early a few days later in compensation. And in order to keep up such a reputation Jo usually covered the extra hours herself. Nor was she a stay-comfortably-in-the-office-with-the-paperwork sister. The rhythmic movement of the bus, took her back there now. Emptying bedpans - holding her breath while she peered at the stools for traces of altered blood. Fighting the nausea as she measured the flecked sputum at

7.30 am - glad she hadn't bothered with breakfast. Feeling the cold slipperiness of all those false teeth as she scrubbed, disinfected, steeped.

How she revelled in the responsibility of her own first ward. The freedom to set the pace and the standards excited her. She was everywhere. Nothing happened but she knew about it. And her standards - well, they were legendary. The stores would be stacked that way - it was more efficient. No, she didn't allow newspapers on the beds without protection - blackened sheets looked so unhygienic - no need for that. Sorry, no more than two visitors at a time - patients were in for a rest - too many visitors, it just tired them. They soon learned - yes, she was a stickler for order and tidiness. They had to fit in with her efficient system.

The back injury she sustained had been a cruel blow. It had been a frantically busy day. Five major operations, two deaths and the collapse of a man who was well on the road to recovery but suddenly developed a pulmonary embolism. Jo was in her element. Rushing here, there, everywhere - adjusting drips, taking blood pressures, giving painkillers, totting up the fluid balance, bathing, listening - well, listening? - just when she had the time. Mr Murray - they'd sent him back from Recovery Room a bit too soon. The vomit went everywhere - needed a complete bed change. She was acutely conscious of the need to save time. An armful of clean linen collected on the way to the sluice for the bucket and mop, that would leave time to see why Mr Braithwaite's catheter wasn't draining properly.

She felt the sickening pain as she went down, heel skidding on the wet floor from a carelessly slopped washing bowl. Instinctively she grabbed for something as she went - the trolley loaded with piles of linen fell on top of her. Oh the mortification of the creased, damp stained uniform. The nurses on duty - offering to help - she didn't want help - far too much work to be done - just get on and get the place sorted out before the visitors arrived. But the pain! The least movement, agony. It must be severe bruising - a few days taking it a bit easier - it'd go.

But it didn't go. It got worse. Two weeks flat on your back, the GP said, and don't put a foot to the floor in that time. Still no improvement. The orthopaedic department next - well, they saw these sorts of things all the time. They'd know. It would have been easier to accept if she'd had a firm diagnosis. Something with a specific name sounded so much more acceptable. Strained muscles - torn ligaments - horribly reminiscent of the language of the malingerer. She would fight on - not for her such a pitiful role. Exercises. Physiotherapy. Manipulation. Heat treatment. Lotions. Massage. Acupuncture. Temporary relief but nothing lasted. Try as she might she just couldn't do the lifting, bending, hurrying. How she hated admitting defeat. But work was - well, an ordeal. So much of what she was so good at was now beyond her. She knew she'd changed - turned from a sparkling enthusiastic leader of her ward team into a grumpy frustrated office administrator. The suggestion came from her GP. Go to work with babies - they aren't so heavy. Reluctantly she considered the option. She had little choice but to give it a try.

Becoming a student again had been harder for Jo than for most. Felt like an endurance test - those sloppy management styles of other ward sisters; having her work checked - hers! Having her ability questioned. How it galled. Younger people than she were the experts. Gritting her teeth, hearing their criticisms, their frustrations with her slowness. And her own anxiety, that oppressed her too. A catastrophic experience at the beginning of her spell in the Neonatal Unit had only underlined her fear.

The houseman - nice young man - Dr Allan - Charles Allan - lovely manner - made you feel you counted. He'd drawn up the intravenous drugs for the sickest babies - laid the syringes on the top of the incubators ready for the treatment round. They all knew this was the routine. It meant the doctor could perform several tasks with each baby rapidly. No unnecessary delays washing hands, assembling equipment. Much less disturbance for the babies.

They needed their time to rest, recover from the frequent insults. But this day - it was evening time - one of the students - Bernice Tarrant her name was, she'd never forget that - Bernice had thought they were oral drugs. Shot them down the tube with the milk. Charles, he'd looked so puzzled. Remembered drawing up the drugs. Definitely. Only baby in the Unit on exactly that combination. The sister in charge, she was puzzled too. No, she hadn't moved them. She checked the charts. BT? Whose signature was it on the feed chart? Bernice Tarrant. First step. Ask her. Had she seen them? Seemed to be the only person who'd seen to the baby since the syringes had been put on the top of the incubator.

Bernice - poor kid - went a whiter shade of ashen. Couldn't cope with the thought of what she'd done. Didn't wait for reassurance. Didn't wait even to check the baby'd be OK. Left that minute - the shift, the Unit, left nursing - for good. There was a distinct air of tragedy over the place.

Lasted several days. Roger had to be consulted. He'd come in immediately to assess the baby. He'd been so gentle and understanding. The shocked sister in charge had burst into tears herself - just because he'd been so nice about it. The infant, he'd been fine, neither up nor down. But the staff, they'd suffered - as much about the blighting of a promising career as the fear for the baby's welfare.

It was all the frustration of feeling personally inadequate that made Jo's rest uneasy on the bus trundling out to Tamforth. Physical weariness was inevitable after eight hours in the intense heat of the Unit, on her feet constantly. On the shifts where she assisted one of the trained staff she felt more at ease, secure in the knowledge that they would notice if she got something wrong. But today there had been no time for doubling up on tasks. She had simply had to pull her weight. It grieved her that the qualified staff seemed not to understand that even the simplest tasks could seem terrifying to a novice like herself. She could only be glad that all her charges had been still alive at the end of her ministrations. Criteria had become very basic.

On top of the frustration though today there was another heaviness. That battle with Wendy Greenaway - it had left her feeling low. She wasn't quite sure why. The passing hedges blurred as she analysed the events. To begin with she hadn't meant to continue the discussion outside the Unit meeting. She'd said her piece. But Wendy had approached her in the changing room.

'I'm really sorry to hear about your nephew,' Wendy's voice was quiet, sounded like she cared. She would though - wouldn't she. Thought they were all so special.

'Thanks - but it would be better if you thought about my sister,' she almost spat out the words. Somehow the Sister's concerned look irritated her - too holy by half. Needed to get her feet on the ground.

'Well, I was thinking of her too ...'

'Doesn't sound like it to me! What do you know - first hand I mean - about bringing up these kids?'

'Well, not as much as you prob ...'

'I know - there is a danger there. And I'm not offering anything - not really. I just wondered if you knew about it. It's up to you, of course. I'm not pressing anything.'

'Well, it's not up to me. It's up to my sister. She gets really fed up - people poking their noses in - stirring things up. Then they go away leaving her to mop up the mess. I'll see. I might tell her about it - depends. I might not. She's sort of getting used to Greg not being able to do anything. It might be too cruel - too cruel to even hint at the possibility of something better.'

'I understand that. Well, I'll leave it with you. But if you change your mind, just let me know.' Wendy turned to leave.

'OK. And - well - thanks.' The words were dragged out reluctantly.

'You're welcome. I'm sorry if what I said - earlier, I mean, upset you. Wasn't my intention.'

'S'OK.'

How Jo regretted her hot temper, her unwillingness to admit she had been at fault. Her desperate need always to be right, to set the standard, now worked against her. Deep down she knew that Wendy had acquitted herself far more creditably. She hadn't won the argument - no-one had - but she had behaved courteously, generously.

The mile-long walk from the bus stop livened her up and she deliberately forced herself to concentrate on admiring the gardens she passed, the sounds of birds chirruping cheerfully all around her. Years of experience had taught her that she simply couldn't take her problems into her sister's house. Unless she got rid of some of her own preoccupation and tension, she'd be in no state to listen to Val.

As she turned into the housing estate where her sister lived, Jo was nearly knocked down by the rush of young bodies playing football. They scarcely noticed her as they shrieked advice to their team mates and abuse at their opponents. She squeezed herself into the hedge as they cavorted wildly around the ball until some ill-judged kick sent it careering along the street and the whole gathering hurtled as one body in hot and noisy pursuit. No. 14 was certainly one of the most disreputable gardens in the road she noted with some dismay. Not that Val had inherited her own obsession with order. It was simply that this was a task she could have helped with - if she'd thought.

The peeling green paint of the front door had been sanded recently and the vigorous hand had revealed evidences of the former red, black and grey leaving a contour map of previous preference. At her ring it opened a few inches and the tousled head and bleary eyes of her sister showed that she had been dozing. The stark contrast between the sisters set them at a distance initially. Jo was tall and slim with sleek brown hair neatly cut in a bob around her unlined face. Her whole outfit today down to the large silk scarf knotted loosely round her shoulders, was carefully matched and toned, all navy blue and white.

Val, two years her senior, looked at least a decade older. Shorter and plumper than Jo, she wore her ginger hair permed into tight curls which poured around her shoulders now where they had escaped the normally restraining combs. The extreme fairness of complexion which so often accompanies red hair had faded to a weary greyness and the amber eyes were heavily circled. Her crumpled jade shirt jarred with the emerald cord trousers and the worn pink slippers completed the picture of defeat.

The two women embraced briefly before Val led the way into the living room. With a deft movement a pile of discarded papers was whisked from the settee, the worst of the crumbs flicked off on to the tired shag pile, absorbed into the greater untidiness. Jo took the proffered seat while Val busied herself gathering the assorted coffee mugs littering the room.

'How are things, Val?' Jo enquired, inching her frame into a dip in the settee.

'Much the same as ever.' The response was automatic.

'Greg - how's he been lately?'

'More cantankerous than ever,' Val was tight-lipped.

Jo was used to this difficult period which characterised her visits initially. Val seemed to have so much anger bottled up - she always projected a hostile image for the first half-hour of their meeting.

'Coffee? Or do you want one of those herbal teas you're so keen on?'

Jo swallowed a sharp retort and asked for coffee. Her every instinct was to wrap her sister in her arms and mother her. It should be the other way round - she should be making the coffee for Val; cooking her a tempting meal. But she knew her sister well after over 30 years. Such good intentions would certainly be misconstrued. She resisted the impulse. The unnecessary banging of cupboard doors made her sigh and resign herself to a frosty conversation until the thaw set in.

The coffee when it came in a thick yellow mug was too milky for her taste but she accepted it without comment.

'Thanks, Val, I'm ready for this. Fell asleep on the bus coming here and my mouth tastes foul.'

'You tired then? Were you working today?' Val's brusque tone seemed to dismiss any right to tiredness Jo might claim.

'Yes, and it was fearfully busy. I was scared to death!'

'Scared? You? You're kidding me!'

'No, honestly. These tiny babies - they petrify me. And I'm dead scared all the time in case I do something wrong - harm them in some way.'

'Isn't there someone else - someone who knows - someone you can ask?'

'Oh, yes, the place is hotching with trained staff. But when it's busy, they simply haven't the time to spend watching us students. You just have to get on with things as best you can. OK, they look after the ventilators and stuff like that - you know, the complicated things. But even feeding these miniscule creatures - it's a nightmare. I stand there, you know -holding the syringe of milk and staring at them to make sure they don't go blue or something equally horrible.'

'Well, it sounds odd - hearing you saying you're out of your depth! I always think that's my problem but you - you're always so - well - so together - so much in control of things.'

'That's all a facade! Inside I'm a quivering wreck. But me - I'm just too proud to show it!' Jo laughed as she spoke, relieved to have a warmer reception.

'Well, I've know you too long and too well to believe that. But I can quite see why you'd be a bit scared - scared of those really tiny ones - at first anyway. At least when you ran your own ward, the patients were adult - pretty tough - able to tell you how they felt. Looking after the prems - well, must be a bit like being a vet. They can't tell you what they're feeling. You feel horribly responsible.'

'Exactly! And you know all the time you couldn't replace one of those wee souls if you did make a cock up.'

A sudden noise above their heads made both women jump. Val seemed to sag in her seat, a look of unutterable weariness on her face.

'He's woken up,' her tone was flat.

'I'll go,' said Jo jumping to her feet. 'Has he been asleep long?'

Val glanced at the clock on the wall.

'All of half an hour,' she sighed. 'But it's probably as well he's awake now - otherwise he wouldn't sleep tonight.'

'D'you want him bringing downstairs or what?' Jo enquired as she moved towards the door.

'Well, yes, I usually do bring him down for tea. But you'd better watch your back. I'll come and give you a hand.' Val reluctantly uncurled herself from the chair and followed her sister up the stairs.

Jo marvelled again at the striking good looks of her nephew - thick dark wavey hair, his mother's huge amber eyes. His adolescent frame had become gauntly angular as he began to leave childhood behind him. The wild spastic movements of his limbs flailing the air aimlessly necessitated a cautious approach. As he caught sight of his aunt he refocused his gaze and slowly a broad grin spread over his face. Deep guttural sounds escaped revealing his pleasure at her visit. Jo inched closer and caught one windmilling arm in her grasp holding it still against her body as she looked into his eyes and said softly,

'Hi there, Greggy. How are things?'

Even wilder gesticulations and a dull roar of sound from deep within told her that he was making a desperate effort to reply.

'We're going to take you downstairs for tea, OK?' Jo asked, still holding one arm firmly as she bent to take the weight of his body before transferring him to a chair.

'Here, watch it!' Val's voice was sharp. She knew from bitter experience how unwieldy her son was to move and Jo's back would not take the strain that she had become accustomed to as Greg had grown bigger and heavier and less cooperative. She nudged her sister to one side and bent her smaller frame to take the sudden onslaught as she expertly manoevred him into the wheelchair. To spare her careworn sister some strain, Jo set to strapping him into the chair before wheeling it out on to the landing and bumping it step by step downstairs. She felt her back rebelling at each jolt but steeled herself to preserve a blank expression. Once he was in the living room Greg became excited again, flailing and grunting in response to his aunt's attempts to converse with him.

Val had disappeared into the kitchen once they were safely downstairs and Jo could hear her noisily crashing utensils and splashing water. The fragrance of grilling bacon made her realize how hungry she was.

'Smells good, eh, Greggy? This one of your favourites?'

His excitement continued but as ever Jo could not possibly differentiate one movement from another, one grunt from another. Only his broad smile seemed to indicate his emotions were positive. What must it be like to be trapped in a body which did nothing to order? Wanting to communicate but absolutely unable to convey a single meaningful word? She often wondered just how alert his mind was. It would be intolerable if he was as sensitively aware as any other normal teenage boy. Who could know.

She continued to chatter on about everything she thought might conceivably interest him until Val reappeared with a bowl of greenish grey slops and a child's plastic bib with a deep pocket for catching spilled food. Val dumped a large apron in Jo's lap with a muttered, 'Better put this on,' before passing her the rest of the load. Jo took the equipment from her, donned the proffered apron and fastening the bib round Greg's neck, proceeded to feed him the thick savoury mix.

'What's in it, Val?' she called out to her sister who had returned to the kitchen.

'Bacon, sausages, potato, peas and beans,' came the answer above the sound of renewed sizzling.

'Scrummy,' Jo put as much delight into the word as she could, hunching her shoulders and screwing up her face as if savouring the food with him.

A random movement of his right arm narrowly missed the dish and she moved smartly to avoid a catastophe. His enjoyment of the food was evident in his ready opening of his mouth for each spoonful. But his control was too poor to enable him to coordinate swallowing and the greenish fluid oozed between his teeth, pouring down the plastic apron even as he gulped each fraction of a spoonful. As she shovelled it back up and fed it again and again, Jo's heart went out as ever to his mother having this task to face three times each day, every day of every week in every year. Endless. Thankless. So ugly.

She glanced ruefully at her own clothes. The apron had shielded her partially but it would take a full protective outfit to prevent the spluttered food from such a radius finding a mark. She felt deeply ashamed of her earlier inner distaste of the squalor in which her sister lived. How could she have thought even for an instant that such superficial things were important. Easy for her in the orderliness of her solitary living to expect neatness and cleanliness as her right; to revel in the coordination of colour and shape - pristine, untrammelled.

When Val returned to check on their progress, Jo felt embarrassed by the mess she and Greg had created between them. In all her years of training and of feeding patients she had never learned the secret as expertly as her sister who had simply been a mother to this severely disabled boy. She resisted the strong temptation to hand the spoon to Val and persevered with the effort to get some nourishment into Greg. Val said nothing about her ineptitude but went to put her meal to keep warm.

Something made Jo ask, 'Val, how do you manage so much better with this job? Why do I make such a dog's dinner of it?'

Val was startled. The second time today her strong competent younger sister had relaxed her guard and admitted she had feet of clay.

'Years of practice, I guess. That's all,' she responded in an expressionless voice. 'And being the one who has to clear up the mess!'

'Well, I wish I had half your expertise and half your patience,' Jo's eyes were on the greenish liquid rushing from Greg's clenched teeth as he hissed through a mouthful sending it everywhere, so she missed the puzzled look her sister shot her.

'Why don't you go ahead - have your meal in peace now while it's fresh?' Jo asked, removing the bowl far from the range of Greg's flailing arms, before glancing at her sister perched warily on the arm of a nearby chair.

'OK, I'll have mine and then take over there while you have yours - if you're sure you want to continue?'

'Sure, I'm sure. You just look away from the mess I make. I'll clear it all up afterwards.' Jo gave Greg her full attention once more. When her sister was settled at the table with her grill, she brought the conversation round to their mother who had recently moved house. Present reflection moved into past and they were soon reminiscing about their childhood, laughing at memories shared of happier carefree days.

Jo continued the mechanical motions of feeding and collecting the dribbles but she was less tense now that she and Val were back on their old footing once more. The tight frown and taut body language had eased and Val was relaxing sloppily over the table as they talked. Having accomplished her task with the first course to the best of her limited ability, she got up and went to the kitchen for the face flannel and towel kept ready for cleaning Greg up after a meal. It took all her strength to hold both his hands still enough to wipe them free from the pervasive stickiness before she settled herself to give him a bowl of chocolate dessert. As the greeny mess was replaced by brown, she wondered idly why Val chose such mucky colours. But Greg's evident love of chocolate was answer enough. It was difficult enough to coordinate a quick dash for his mouth between flails when he wanted the food; it would be impossible to give him something he disliked.

By the time she had finished feeding Greg the dessert, Val had scraped her plate clean, so she took over giving the additional fluids while Jo went to clean herself up. It was good to have food prepared for her but somehow the battle with the liquidised slops had robbed Jo of her earlier appetite and it was a struggle to eat the bacon and sausages.

This time she made her own coffee. She leaned back in her chair letting the thick, dark bitter fragrance repair her frayed edges. Val had switched on the television set, and she too was silent, intently watching the news. Greg's moans and grunts were subdued and a temporary peace settled on the strangely ill-assorted group.

When Jo rose to go to the kitchen to clear up, Val yawned, stretching expansively, the movement dislodging her shirt, revealing her midriff. Jo tried to encourage her to rest while she did the washing-up but Val was insistent that she dried up and put things away. She knew her sister's propensity to rearrange her kitchen. There would be a major reshuffle - an attempt to make everything logical. It would take her twice as long to accomplish her tasks until everything was once again in its familiar place. Their chatter was of superficial interests and a comfortable air of familiarity facilitated a smooth transition from one subject to another. Even so, Jo threatened their amicable exchange in one unguarded move. Having washed up, she proceeded automatically to clean the surfaces. A blistering rebuke from Val awoke her to the perceived criticism of her level of cleanliness. Protests fell on stubbornly deaf ears and it took all Jo's persuasive powers to jolly her older sister back into communication.

It was then time to prepare Greg for bed. With visits from her sister so infrequent, Val elected to forgo a full bath for him - but yes, if she insisted Jo could do the honours. Rigidly flexed limbs made even undressing him a feat. Lurching for a hand or a foot between wildly spastic jerks, Jo wondered if this was an indication that this developing young man resented such invasion of his privacy. Or was it simply that as the clothes were removed there was less to restrain the limbs. She was back with the babies - the normal babies - no hint of spasticity - they startled and quivered when you unwrapped them, laid them naked on a sheet. How much more reason for grotesque contortions here! How many 13-year-olds were so crudely exposed to the eyes of mother and aunt? How many teenagers were so powerless to protect themselves from unwanted attentions? Nappy changing reinforced her sense of his potential embarrassment and she was less than thorough in her cleansing. His mother had no such scruples, however, and pushed her aside to remedy the fumbling deficiencies.

'For goodness sake! Call yourself a nurse? He'll be sore within 12 hours if you don't clean him up properly!' she growled applying herself to the task with more energy than sensitivity.

She was right of course, Jo mused. But on this occasion she had allowed her feelings as a woman and an aunt to overcome her usual detachedness. Not for the first time she thought how much more sensibly Val had coped with disablement than she would ever have done. Or did you just adapt from sheer necessity? Her own inate love of beauty, order, neatness seemed to make everything so much harder to accept. But perhaps Val too would have loved such things if circumstances had been different.

In his blue pyjamas, hair and face free from the remnants of his battle with food, Greg looked younger and less fiercely resistant. As his mother expertly scrubbed his clenched teeth he even managed to cooperate with rinsing and spitting sufficiently to avoid her altogether. And once in bed when she leaned down to kiss him goodnight he held still and rubbed his cheek gently against hers for a brief moment of gentle appreciation.

Jo had volunteered to read to him from the current bedtime book and settled herself in the wicker chair beside him so that the circle of light from the lamp fell brightly on her page but avoided his wide eyes. She knew from the absence of grunting that he was listening and she was surprised at the flood of warm pleasure it gave her to be giving him something meaningful. She renewed her efforts to make the story live for him. It had been a source of wonder to her that Val always retained this habit of a quiet time reading to her son, no matter how grim the day or how weary her body. Now she, an infrequent aunt, was reaping the rewards of this selfless devotion. She was tempted to extend the regulation two chapters, to give him a little treat which he might associate with her visit, but a stronger reluctance to antagonise her sister made her close the book and explain her going. Of late she had wondered whether it was appropriate still to embrace this young man. If he were normal he would probably keep well out of arms length. She found herself telling Greg of her dilemma, appealing to him to let her know by some means when she did things which he didn't like. The flailing and the grunting were indecipherable so she dropped a brief kiss on her moving target, assured him she'd be back again soon, switched off the light and left him to his unfathomable world.

For once relieved of a task, Val had settled down with the newspaper to await Jo's return. Within minutes she was sound asleep. Jo stood looking down at the prematurely aged woman with compassion. How delicate her features were in repose, softer without the tight frown. The tumbled red curls were still lustrous, the figure still firm and shapely beneath its strident clothing. Free from the tension of Val's prickliness, Jo allowed her eyes to see beyond the careworn image to the girl she might have been.

She saw again the beautiful sister of 14 years ago she herself remembered with such clarity.

What a stunning girl Val had been in her late teens. Not for her the years of puppy fat, the adolescent pimples, the shy awkwardness of departing childhood. The other girls, they were all desperate to keep her favour and friendship. The boys were all crazy about her. Val was never without an escort. How her gawky, angular younger sister had envied her - her curves, her poise, her popularity. Many a night Jo had cried herself to sleep, unable to bear the comparison. And it wasn't just her looks. She'd been brainy too. OK, not as able as Jo herself - but she'd got provisional places at two universities. Seemed to have an easy knack of combining sufficient study with a crowded social life. The parents, they'd worried - concerned about the endless round of dates and parties. But somehow she seemed never to feel tired - was endlessly good-humoured. Until August 13th. Jo remembered it clearly. Their mother's birthday. The whole family had gone out for a meal to celebrate. Val wasn't herself. Three times she'd left the table - precipitately - rushed to the ladies' cloakroom.

Mother, she'd been so concerned. It spoiled her birthday. She worried Val had caught some kind of a bug. They'd left the hotel early, and Val was despatched to bed. Warm soothing drinks, thermometers, pungent gargles - Mother applied all the remedies Grandma had instilled into her. Jo remembered her mother's increasing concern. The vomiting persisted. The bloom left Val's cheeks. Fasting, that eased the ferocity of the sickness. But the nausea was so severe, any smell of food brought on the body-wracking retching. Mother didn't readily admit defeat in the care of her family's health. But after two weeks, she overrode Val's protests, and made an appointment for her to see the doctor. Val insisted she'd go on her own - didn't need to be molly coddled.

It was a week later. She'd seen Mother coming out of Val's room, ashen face. Looked like she was going to faint, leaning on the wall outside to hold herself up. Not a bit like Mother. Eyes closed, hands clenched, gulping great drafts of airs.

'Mum! What's wrong? Are you ill?' Jo had rushed to her aid.

But Mother had shrugged off her hand. Looked at her - didn't seem to see her. Like a stranger. Jo had recoiled from the frozen face.

'I'm all right. Just leave me in peace.' She'd groped her way into her own bedroom, shut the door - hard. Keep out.

Jo had been so frightened, bewildered. She'd flung herself unheralded into her sister's room. Val was lying there, curled up like those pictures of fetuses, all in a bunch on the patchwork, staring vacantly at the window.

'Val, what's wrong with Mum? Is she ill? She looks awful!' The words tumbled out because of her great love for her mother - because of this unknown tragedy that had befallen them.

'She'll be all right.' Val mumbled into her arms, shielding her face. Jo couldn't read her expression. What kind of a response was that - she'd be all right?

'But what's wrong with her?' She heard her voice wailing in her fear.

'You're too young to understand. Just leave her alone.' Why was everyone shutting her out?

Beside herself, she'd sprung to the bed, shaken her sister.

'I'm not too young! I know she's ill. I saw. Tell me! Tell me! Is she dying?'

Something of her terror seemed to reach through to Val - at last. She rolled over. Of course, it was Jo's imagination again, running rampant, giving her nightmares. She'd never understood it but she knew the fears were real - to Jo. What a state she got herself into!

Now Val propped herself up on one elbow, flung the other arm round the heaving shoulders.

'Don't be such an idiot, Jo! Mum's OK. You do get yourself so worked up about nothing!'

Nothing! It didn't feel like nothing!

Over the years, since she was four, Jo had dreaded so many things - things that had never materialised. Could this be just another such figment of an overactive imagination? Val was telling her so, wasn't she? Nothing to worry about. But she felt uneasy - vaguely. Val didn't quite meet her eyes.

No more insight from this encounter was forthcoming. Jo withdrew. It was not easy being 15 and surrounded by people who thought you were still a child. She'd flounced back into her own room, started to play her latest tape loudly - anything to drown out the rest of the world's unkindness.

Over the next few weeks the uneasiness would not be suppressed. The sudden cessations of conversations, the closed doors, her parents raised voices late at night - they all told an unknown story. Now Val stayed at home, locked in her own room with her own private thoughts. No more staying out late with an endless stream of friends.

It was a full five weeks after she had seen her mother's shock before Jo dared to voice her new dread. Her mother had come into her room to remind her of the lateness of the hour. She had approached Jo at her desk, dropped a quick kiss on her head, peered over her shoulder at the detailed drawing of the circulatory system Jo had spent all evening perfecting.

'Still bent on a career in medicine or nursing, eh?'

'I just love all this stuff we're doing in biology, Mum. Do you think this is any good?'

'It's fantastic, darling. Easy to see you love that subject.'

Suddenly, before her courage deserted her, Jo blurted out her question.

'Mum, is Val terribly ill? Is she going to die?' She whirled round in her seat as she spoke, the better to detect a lie. She noted with sick dread the closed expression which came over her mother's face, the defeated look in every line as she sagged on to the bed. For a long moment it looked as if she wouldn't share the secret. But then she had seemed to focus on the terror struck face - gathered her in her arms. Jo felt the rigidness. It must be bad.

'Oh, my poor baby! I had no idea you thought that!' Mother was soothing her, stroking her. Denying it - over and over again.

'Well, what is wrong with her then? I hear her being sick all the time - she doesn't go out. She used to be out all the time. She had to go to the doctor. You go in her room - close the door - whisper to her. And you and Dad - you get cross more than you used to. She won't tell me - anything. And I thought ... I thought ...' She couldn't bring herself to articulate her mortal fear.

She was totally unprepared for the truth. Biology might be her favourite subject but then, aged 15, her knowledge of life had been pretty rudimentary. Val couldn't be having a baby! How could she? What about going to university? Why...? How...? What...? When...? The questions tumbled out in wild confusion. She dimly felt her mother's pain but her own desperate need for information forced her to persist. It was incomprehensible. Was she going to get married and have her own home instead of going to study and have a good time?

Mother had found it so hard to explain that no she wasn't going to get married; she was going to try to get a flat of her own and bring the baby up alone. Jo's incomprehension reflected her own astounded response. Years later she had explained it all. She couldn't accept that her beloved, protected daughter had got herself into such a mess. The world had lain at her feet. Thoughtless abandon, careless disregard, blind youthful passion - call it what you would, she had wilfully thrown away her reputation, her moral principles, her whole future. Or so it seemed to her distraught mother. Dad, he had closed himself off - it was the only way. They knew how he idolised them - both of his daughters - worshipped them. He could not let himself dwell on this outward demonstration that his little girl had left him and given herself to some other fellow - a chap he'd never met - an immature, selfish lout no doubt, concerned only for his personal gratification and hang the consequences. Mother, when she needed him most, found him unavailable to her. He could hardly bear to be in the same room as Val. It was down to Mother - as ever - to comfort, to guide, to present the options. She'd had to respect Val's dogged refusal to name the father of her child. She had to be partner, parent, counsellor - all rolled into one. She was oppressed by the responsibility. It had helped - just a little - helped to share it with Jo, so like her father in many ways.

The months had dragged slowly by. Val's pregnancy became an open secret. Jo hated the nudges, the sniggers, the inuendoes at school. She withdrew more and more into herself - building a protective crust few could penetrate. She spent increasing periods of time in her own room seeking solace in her study. Mother began knitting, buying tiny items. Dad grew more silent, less demonstrative with them all. Val herself had ever more frequent trips to clinics, classes and the housing agencies. Her youthful curves were lost in the unshapeliness of maternity clothes. Something more than her childhood playmate was lost to the bewildered Jo.

It was during the seventh month of the pregnancy that Jo had awoken to a comotion in the adjacent room. Val lay still, rigid, withdrawn, in a pool of liquor as her mother frantically rushed around phoning the hospital and the ambulance service, stuffing clothes into bags. The paramedics were calm and so matter-of-fact they made her mother look hysterical. As suddenly they had gone. A frightening silence settled over the house. It was 2am - frosty - January cold. Jo and her father huddled together for warmth and comfort, afraid - so afraid of something unknown, unwanted.

Each phone call added further to their fears. Dad was summonsed at 6am. His face had looked so gaunt, so old. His voice was hoarse.

'Now, you are going to have to be very brave.'

Clutching at his arm she had insisted that she go too. She might only be 15 but she was old enough to face a family tragedy with them. Looking back at that time she had only dimly understood the fight for her sister's life. She heard words like 'fits'... 'blood pressure through the roof'... 'terminate the pregnancy'... 'slim chance' through a haze of terror and her mother's sobbing. Greg had been born a puny little purple creature - more like a skinned rabbit than a baby boy. It all felt so unreal - seeing him through a porthole in the door of a single room. If she pinched herself would she wake up to another regular school morning? She didn't dare pinch herself in case the reality was worse than her nightmare. They hadn't let her even see her sister for four days; they said she needed absolute quiet and darkness. Her mother stayed in the hospital each night to be on hand in case ... In case of what? When she did finally visit, Val's appearance had scared Jo more than any anticipated change. She looked bloated somehow, white skin puffed around dazed eyes, red hair damply matted to her head, coarse hospital gown stained with leaking milk. Jo's tongue stuck to her dry palate. There were no words in their teenage vocabulary to bridge the chasm that had yawned between them over those few days.

Gradually the old Val re-emerged in appearance. But something of her youth had gone for ever. Anxiety for her baby - Val's baby - sounded so odd, Val's baby - battling for his life in the special nursery, etched deep lines around her eyes. Hours she spent - simply sitting beside his incubator, willing him to keep breathing, totally preoccupied with him.

Then there were the endless trips to the hospital - weeks and weeks after her own discharge home. No, her soulmate had gone for ever.

It was five months before Greg was finally allowed to come home. And now even greater changes disturbed the old order. Val became an obsessive mother, hyper anxious, fraught by the persistent screeching cry, worn down by the endless frustration of trying to get enough feeds into a reluctant child. Mother hovered between supportive aide and over protective grandmother. Val was still only 18, unversed in the ways of motherhood. But this was her baby, Val protested, her mother's views and practices were out of date now! The friction grew. Tension spilled over into the other areas of their daily living, drawing Jo and her father unwillingly into the foray. Finally an escalation of hostility over a night feed drove Val to seek a flat alone with her son. The Council housed her in an undesirable neighbourhood, but at least she could close her own door to interfering good intentions.

Hurt and excluded, Val's parents kept away. Jo's visits were short and uneasy - Val seemed to be holding on by the skin of her teeth. She remembered again the shock - that day when she'd gone and found a man there, holding the baby. Phil had moved in with Val. So, she preferred a stranger to her own family, did she? No, Val explained, it wasn't like that. She'd known Phil for years at school and they had had a brief tumultuous romance in fifth year. A chance meeting in the supermarket had renewed the acquaintance and Val had been so grateful for his company during the long solitary vigils between feeds. His visits became more frequent. It became a practical advantage to share accommodation. They took it in turns to cook, clean, shop, change and feed Greg. They settled down into a vaguely uncertain rut. But when Val's parents eventually met him, they had, grudgingly, to admire his dexterity with their grandson.

It had been Mother who had first, tentatively suggested that Greg was not growing quite as she would expect. Val was furious, storming out of the house with her precious baby, stung by her mother's perspicacity. But she'd had her own doubts. They wouldn't be stilled. When the health visitor recommended more tests she'd reluctantly agreed. Recognition of the extent of the damage had been slow. What was a slight backwardness in an infant became an obvious deficit and then a social embarrassment as he matured and failed to acquire control or independence. A chronic air of sorrow aged his mother inch by inch as she struggled to come to terms with a dawning reality. Phil developed grim lines around his mouth and began working late night after night.

When he finally declared he could take no more, Val withdrew into a silent world of bitter sadness. Mother was ready to come out of the wings where she had stood guardedly for eight years. Greg was still her grandson. She loved him in spite of all the hurt and all the hopelessness. And so it was that the family regrouped, repairing as best they could the breaches and the betrayals. The grandparents had the patience Val lacked. They would spend hours coaxing the rebellious child to feed or dress. But Greg grew rapidly and became too large and ungainly for Mother's arthritic joints.

She had to content herself with undertaking the domestic chores; freeing Val up for the daily relentless battles with her son.

When Dad had died - suddenly, unexpectedly - Greg was 11. Without his chauffeuring, Mother's visits became less frequent. Jo's busy career, her back injury, limited her involvement. Val was forced to shoulder the burden alone. She had been more hurt than she cared to admit by Phil's defection. He had been a beacon of hope on her bleak horizon. Having someone to share both the regular grim troubles and the brief respite hours had been some solace. Her bottled anger and low self-esteem made her more than ever volatile. Jo found her hostile moods wearing. You needed to be pretty robust to pay a visit these days.

Now she looked down at the sleeping form with deep pity. What a raw deal life had dealt this potentially beautiful woman. Only her fierce love for her son redeemed her pitiful situation. Stirred by the deep lines of fatigue, Jo crept away into the kitchen and set to work preparing a pot of soup ready for the following day. One less task in her sister's grossly overworked life.

It was a good hour before Val awoke to the fragrance of leeks cooking. She staggered drunkenly to the kitchen, muttering apologies for her unsociable behaviour and protests at her sister working in her time off. Only half awake she brewed a pot of tea and the two sat on the kitchen stools idly chatting about mundane affairs. When they both called in to check on

Greg they were giggling together about a remembered incident in their childhood, repressing the sound so as not to wake the sleeping boy.

The sight which greeted their eyes stifled any desire to laugh. Excrement smeared over walls and bedding framed the flailing form in the bed. The stench made the two women recoil.

For one electric moment they stood open mouthed taking in the scene. The wild eyes of the tormented boy roamed the room passing them without recognition. Jo was totally unprepared for what happened next. Val galvanised into action leapt towards him and began hammering her fists on to his body. A venomous string of expletives issued through clenched teeth. Her shaking of the spastic form further spread the filthiness all around him. It took all Jo's strength to extricate her sister from the violence which rained down on the helpless boy. Holding her arms in a vice-like grip she shouted at Val to be quiet and forced the shaking form into a nearby chair.

'Sit there and get a grip on yourself, d'you hear me? Don't you move until I tell you you can. I'll start stripping the bed and clear up the walls and so on and then you can help me with the turning and the bit that needs both of us. OK? SIT .. THERE .. AND .. DON'T .. MOVE!'

As suddenly as it had come, the anger dissipated and Val shrank back defeated in the chair. Apparently oblivious to her soiled hands she wrapped her arms around her hunched up knees and rocked herself back and forth in miserable abjection. Jo set to work stripping the soiled linen, and bowls of steaming water liberally laced with Dettol soon brought the situation under control. She managed to strip Greg and wash his besmeared body on her own for once. Was it her imagination, or did he seem cowed, afraid? Could he understand that his mother was in a towering rage - and he was to blame in some way? Jo hoped devoutly he was spared such insight.

Val seemed unaware of what was going on, sitting staring vacantly into space throughout the procedure. Jo's touch was gentle but expert now as she massaged body lotion into the grossly contorted form, soothing him with her low voice as she worked, glad for his sake when fresh pyjamas and coverlet protected his defencelessness. One look at her sister's huddled form had persuaded her against enlisting any help from that quarter. Several changes of water later she had the surrounding areas back to normal and went into the bathroom to sluice the sheets. It was not until the washing machine was destroying the evidence that she approached Val softly. Kneeling in front of her she coaxed her back to reality before escorting her to the bathroom for a shower and change into nightclothes.

Swallowed up in a peach dressing gown, Val sat beside the fire sobbing uncontrollably in her sister's arms. Jo let her weep until her reservoir of hurt was unlocked. The whole story came rushing out, words jostling incoherently at first as the misery and futility of it all was laid bare. The pain went back 14 years to the day Val had realized she was pregnant. She hadn't told the father about the baby - didn't know who the father was even - there'd been more than one boy. At least she didn't know then but as Greg grew up he looked so much like Sean, it had to be his. Too late then to tell him. Any case, no need to blight another life. Mother and Dad - Dad especially - had wanted her to get rid of it, but the more insistent they were the more she dug her heels in. Oh, if only she had listened to their strictures on morality! She'd just thought they were fuddy duddies with old fashioned ideas about virginity. And it might have been better to have had the pregnancy terminated - she probably would have if they hadn't suggested it.

Every stage of Greg's life had been horrendous. Even as a baby he'd been so hard to feed. And always there was that relentless, piercing crying. She'd several times got near to smothering him in his cot just to blot out the screeching. If it hadn't been for Phil she'd have done something desperate years ago, or perhaps just walked out of the house one day and never come back. She did that one day - walked out. But she'd only got to the railway station and just had to go back. Throughout it all, Phil had been so good. He had made her feel like a woman again. She hadn't been able to believe her luck when he had been keen enough to take on someone else's baby too. And he was so patient - just what she needed. Even when Greg kept crying Phil had managed to stay cool and he took charge when she got hysterical. It had hurt, hurt badly when he deserted her. She knew he had had enough of her temper and her wailing about the unfairness of it all. She had driven him away. The guilt didn't soften the blow. When he left she had finally turned her back on any chance of happiness in this life. Nothing left now but caring for her travesty of a son. Oh yes, she loved Greg - loved him fiercely. But the unending slog brought her often to a homicidal state. She wasn't really as strong as they all thought she was. She put on a show. She had her pride too.

Jo listened aghast to this catalogue of failed support. Tears spilled down her own cheeks as she soothed the heaving frame in her arms.

'Oh, Val, I'm so sorry - so very, very sorry. We've all let you down so badly,' she gulped between their combined sobs.

'No, it's my own doing. I knew I was taking a risk - going with boys like that. But because it was forbidden, it - I don't know - added spice to the adventure. I knew Mother and Dad would have a conniption - wouldn't they though? - if they knew. And even though I didn't want to get pregnant, at first I can remember thinking, "Well, now they'll know that I don't have to take any notice of them. I **can** go and do my own thing and they can't really stop me." What a fool! All of this just because I wanted to be grown up and independent.'

The two women talked long into the night, sharing for the first time the full horror of Val's situation. It was only when Val shuddered, 'Sometimes I wish he had never been born,' that Jo's thoughts returned to her present professional dilemma. She moved on the lumpy settee to a position where she could look into her sister's eyes, red rimmed and puffy now from her weeping. Recounting the Flanaghan's story she simplified the details so that Val could understand them in relation to her own experience with Greg.

'So, if you had to advise those parents, Val, what would you tell them?'

'No question! Let him go now. Quit while you're ahead. It might hurt like hell now to lose a baby, but it sure as hell will hurt a whole lot more having to suffer for the rest of your life.' The language and the tone were the old fiery Val.

'You don't mind, do you, that I mentioned you and Greg in the Unit?' Jo was anxious, mindful of Val's uncertain temper. She had no wish to destroy this closeness that had been born of her sister's brokenness. But she felt a need for absolute integrity.

'No, of course not. I think you were very brave to own up to having a severely abnormal relative. Lots of people'd have been too ashamed to admit to it. And if it stops those sanctimonious prats inflicting a 'beautifying experience' on some other unsuspecting souls, all power to your elbow. What drivel! Bring out finer qualities in parents, indeed! Balderdash - absolute balderdash!'

Jo was cheered by the return of some of her old abrasiveness.

'Actually, Val, there's something I specially wanted to tell you - about this Wendy I've been telling you about.'

'Do I want to hear it? Sounds like a holy git to me!'

'Well, I know. My feelings exactly. But it's only fair to tell you what she said - you can decide yourself whether you do anything about it.'

'Well, go on. About what?'

'Well, she used to work in this Home - a Home for severely damaged kids - you know, like Greg. And she reckons that the woman who runs the place - some nun or other - well, this nun knows a place where they can assess the kids and help them do more for themselves.'

Jo paused looking anxiously at her sister for signs of anger at yet another intrusion. But Val was listening, calmly, interested.

'She said she'd get the address if I - if you were interested. I said I'd mention it - didn't give her any definite answer. It's up to you.'

'And d'you think she knows what she's talking about - this Wendy person?'
'Well, much as I hate all her religious stuff, she's a brilliant neonatal nurse. Seems to really understand the babies, you know. And the parents - they all love her. Seek her out specially, you know. She's - well, it's difficult to describe - but she's got something special going with these families. Obviously in the right specialty.'

'Well, if she's that good, maybe it's worth a try. Actually, I've been wondering - lately, you know, well, it seems like sometimes, Greg understands - more than we thought he did - before.'

'And it must be hard to tell - when they're babies - how much they can do - how far they'll develop and everything.'

'Yeah, must be.' Val was quiet, reflective.

'So d'you want me to - shall I ask her - find out ...?'

'Yeah - I s'pose so - nothing to lose.'

Except her pride, Jo thought ruefully, remembering her own ungraciousness. But that was a small price to pay. She too had wondered lately, about Greg and what went on inside that deformed shell.

It was too late now for her to catch the bus home so she borrowed toiletries and a nightie and made up the bed in the spare room. Something made her put her head round Greg's door before retiring. There she found Val leaning over him dropping soft kisses on to his tousled curls. She heard the murmured apologies as the mother acknowledged her offences to the sleeping child. She could never really explain to him her violent outbursts, they bore no relation to the perceived crime. They were simply the outpourings of a heart broken by suffering, a body taxed beyond human endurance. He could never fathom the depths of her bruised soul.

After a night broken by strangely unfinished dreams, Jo made the best of the available offices to smarten up her appearance. She borrowed a dusty pink shirt from her sister, resisting the urge to re-iron its creases. Breakfast was a desultory affair, Jo again attending to feeding Greg, energy for flailing arms and legs restored by his untrammelled deep sleep.

In the midst of this task the door bell heralded an early visitor. Val had recently befriended a woman of uncertain years, Bridget, who entered now with her son, Jason. One look confirmed that this lad who must be much of an age with Greg, suffered from Down's Syndrome. The introductions over, Jason rushed up to Jo threw his arms around her and gave her a crushing embrace which threatened to upset the dish of porridge she held. Bridget looked uncomfortable but merely murmured ineffectually, 'Jason, don't - please!'

The sadness of her whole demeanour touched Jo's heart. What a strange cruel world these women inhabited. Crushed by experience, they had to bear one humiliation upon another - powerlessly, hopelessly, always. She heard Val explain that she was a nurse and she'd understand. Odd how Val had such faith in her professional training. She seemed to think it made her impervious to human feelings. No amount of training could make her comfortable with Jason's exploring hands - chromosomally abnormal he might be but he was still a human male taking unacceptable liberties with her female body. She instinctively rose from her seat and extricated herself with more speed than sensitivity from his clasp.

'Oh, I'm so sorry. He doesn't mean any harm. He's just affectionate,' his mother was stuttering in her embarrassment.

Jo's voice was cool, distant.

'I know. I understand.'

She left the room to warm the rest of Greg's porridge, taking longer in the sanctuary of the shabby kitchen than the simple task dictated. She knew she's been cruel, caring more about her own dignity than this poor woman's comfort. Would Bridget wish that Jason's life had been snuffed out at an early age, she wondered? Oh, you heard so much about the love these Down's children brought to parents' lives. You didn't hear nearly so much about the other side. Still disturbed by the emotions of the preceding evening, from the revelations that had followed so many years of ignorant calm, she felt too tired to think logically. She had an overwhelming desire to escape back to the safety of the Neonatal Unit where professional standards and an impersonal uniform protected you; where strident abnormality was hidden by the immaturity of infancy. She longed for the tranquillity of her own home where no aberrant behaviour could disturb the calm of an ordinary life.

As soon as Greg was fed and changed she took her leave. Guilt gnawed at her even as she hugged her sister warmly, promising to return soon. Easy for her, regulating her contact with tragedy. Easy for Wendy, to say all life is sacred. Easy for her, to commit other parents to a lifetime of misery. Easy for her ... Easy for her ... Easy for her ... The trundling wheels lulled her into sleep as she was carried back to safety.

CHAPTER 6

The Chaplain's Lot

It was late on Thursday evening when the chaplain finally arrived in his office and sank down in his rather shabby chair. It had been a long and draining day.

First there had been the general round of the patients in the areas for which he held a pastoral responsibility. Although aware of the scant interest of most of them in spiritual matters, Martin nevertheless saw his role as bringing comfort in a rather general way. At least he took an interest in each one of them, cared how they were progressing. It never ceased to amaze him how few visitors some patients seemed to get. He hoped he was better than nothing. Being a realist, he strongly suspected that few appreciated any blessing he might pronounce but his dog collar gave him the right to do so where he thought it appropriate.

There had been one very difficult encounter that morning with a young woman of 23 who had a history of drug misuse. She had been in so many times Martin had lost count and he had to some extent become inured to her snide personal comments. But today Melanie was different. She had just been told that she had contracted HIV. It was she who had blurted this out to him amongst a stream of foul language and jibes against life, ministers of a 'useless religion' and God himself. The chaplain knew that counselling always accompanied the disclosure of this particular diagnosis. Neither was he any stranger to the anger which such news generated. But his heart sank as he inwardly recoiled from the hurled abuse of this woman. He had never seen her quite so frenzied. There seemed no way of reaching out to her and yet he felt her abominable behaviour was in some strange way a cry for help.

Martin resisted the strong impulse to escape from her foul invectives. He was glad she was housed in a single room and he made sure the door was quite shut before he took a seat in the chair beside her bed. He schooled himself to say nothing but kept his eyes fixed on her, willing himself to convey to her his concern and compassion. When she had finally exhausted her extensive vocabulary of obscenities, she suddenly slumped back on her pillows and turned her head away from him. Martin remained silent for a long moment offering up a silent prayer for help. Then very quietly he said, 'I am so very, very sorry.'

'Whit d'you care?' Her words sounded so venomous.

'It hurts me to see you hurting so much.'

'Ah'm no hurtin'. Ah'm mad! Ah'm bluidy mad.'

'What are you mad about?'

'Soddin' everythin''

'Especially the HIV?' Martin held his breath. Was his long acquaintance with this girl sufficient to allow him to tread this close to her raw pain?

A choked intake of breath and a shuddering of the thin body inside the purple dressing gown gave him the courage to continue. Perhaps it was as well she kept her eyes averted. At least she couldn't see his uncertainty.

'I'm sure it's horrendous to hear that you've got it, but heaps of people I've talked to have told me that when they've had a bit of time to take it in and they realize they can still have years and years of doing the things they want to do, it doesn't seem quite so awful.' The long silence unnerved him somewhat.

Finally a small voice asked, 'Ye've blethered wi' other folks wi' it?'

'Indeed I have. Many of them.'

'An' are ye no' scared o' bein' near them?'

'No, why should I be?'

'Are ye no' feart o' catchin' it?'

'No.' Martin put as much emphasis into this little negative as he could. 'I won't catch anything from them. In fact I'm probably more of a risk to them than they are to me.'

'Hoo's that then?' Melanie had become very still and Martin felt her absorption in their exchange.

'Well, because they are so much more vulnerable to infections than people usually are and they get more sick if they catch something like a cold.'

'They telt me that,' she appeared to be whispering to herself. 'Bu' hoo d'you ken that?' with this she flung herself round to face him almost accusingly. 'Ye telt me ye was a kinda meenister. Sae hoo d'ye ken things like tha'?'

'Because I try to understand what these things mean for people so I don't get it wrong - say things that won't be helpful. So I ask the doctors and nurses about what different illnesses mean. And sometimes, when I can, I go along to lectures they have on some of the ones I don't know enough about.'

'An' wus it them whit telt ye 'bout me?'

'No, definitely not. No-one is allowed to tell anyone else confidential information about any patient. I only know what you've told me about yourself.'

'Wish Ah'd kep' me bluidy mooth shut!'

'I'm sorry you feel like that because I only want to help.'

'Naebody kin help me noo.' A flounce turned her head away again but not before he saw a tell-tale glisten in her eye.

'They can if you'll let them.'

'Hoo kin they?'

'Well, the nurses and doctors - they can help you to steer away from the things that make you more ill. And there are counsellors to talk to, if you want to try to sort out your feelings. And I'm happy to come and talk with you - if you'd like to try that out.'

She was silent but Martin took heart from the moderated language and her stillness.

'Does Billy know?' Billy was the partner whom Melanie had taken up with after a particularly traumatic spell in a detoxification unit some years earlier. Billy was himself addicted to drugs and it was not long before Melanie was even deeper into her habit than before. Martin had met him once and had no wish to repeat the experience. His language and behaviour made Melanie look almost virtuous.

Now she said simply, 'Ah dinnae stay wi' him noo.'

'Is there anyone else?'

'Naw.'

The sheer loneliness of the figure on the bed made Martin want to reach out and touch her but he resisted the impulse fearing to disturb the quiet rationality of their present exchange.

'Where d'you stay now then?'

'Onywhaur.'

'What about your family? They know where you are?'

'Naw.'

'D'you think you could tell them?'

'Whit d'they care?'

'Because parents usually do care - deep down they do, even if they find it difficult to show you they do.'

'Mebees.'

'Worth a try?' A shrug was her only response.

'Would you like me - or anyone else - to help you to make contact with them? Sometimes it's easier - you know - if you have someone else on your side.'

'Ah'll think aboot it.' Another long pause followed before she murmured almost to herself, 'They'll no' want tae ken noo. Ah wouldnae want tae mysel'.'

'That might depend on how they're told. Once they understand there's absolutely no risk to them, I think you might be surprised at how much people want to help.'

Tears rolled down her blotched cheeks but all she said was, 'Mebees.' Without knowing any more about her family he felt it would be wrong to build her hopes too much but his instinct to convey to this waif that she need not stand alone impelled him to go on.

'I'd be glad to pop in to see you every little while - if you'd like me to, that is. And we can see if there's anything practical we can arrange to help you, when you feel ready to make decisions. Not just yet - just when you're ready.'

'Aye, OK. If ye kin be bothered.'

For answer he touched her hand briefly. She raised startled eyes to his and almost blurted out, 'Ye're no' feart tae touch me?'

'No. Why should I be?'

'Cos Ah've got - got - ye ken!' It was too near the diagnosis for her to be able actually to say the words.

'That doesn't make you a leper! I know when I'm feeling down it helps if someone holds my hand or gives me a hug or something.' Martin held her gaze for a long moment and taking her silence as a good omen he took her hand in a strong clasp.

'You don't have to go it alone. There are lots of people here who'll be only too ready to help you if you'll let them. And things won't seem quite so black in a little while. So hang in there!' His smile was warm and genuine. Since she did not snatch her hand away he was emboldened to add softly, 'God bless you', before he left her to her musing on what he had said. Important not to push her too far too soon.

These encounters were so draining he wanted so much to escape to the peace of his own room. But he was already late for the rest of his visits so he took a big breath and proceeded down the corridor. The next hour passed in a haze. Meg Winston - how she prattled on about her gallstones - as if it was important how big they were and just how nauseated she had been. Jim Darren always had a complaint to confide - the hospital service was never good enough for him. Today it was the laundry in disgrace - they'd run out of drawsheets - had to use paper ones. What did it matter, Martin reflected - the old codger didn't change his sheets every day at home, did he? But he listened dutifully, clucked his tongue in all the right places. Better for him to get the wingeing than the overworked nurses.

Dot Harris was one of the few patients who professed a religious affiliation. Devout Methodist - like her father and his father before him. In the blood. 'Bin gaein' tae chapel since Ah were a bairn.' He felt so uncomfortable with her querulous determination to leave her fate in God's hands. His God didn't act in that kind of direct way. But it helped her to believe she was specially protected. It was no part of his role to shatter illusions. At least not the ones that got people through the bad times. Anyway, who was to say he was right and she was wrong. He had his doubts too. But he preferred Simon Radcliff's robust challenging of a God who allowed hospitals to fill up with sick folk. Radcliffe always tried to stir him up to defend his belief. Today Martin was all too conscious that he had to keep dragging his attention back from Melanie. By comparison with hers, these other problems seemed so trivial. How did you begin to deal with the prospect of your own death - when you were 23? His brief words to most of the patients sounded hollow in his ears but years of practice had made him quite slick with the common courtesies.

It was nearly one o'clock before he finally finished his rounds of the adult wards in 'his patch' as he termed it. There was just time for a quick sandwich before he had to dash out and collect his aged mother and ferry her across town for a clinic appointment. He wanted to appear bright and cheerful for her. She only worried about him if he seemed downcast and he was scrupulous about not taking confidences out of the hospital for others to share. His could be a lonely job at times.

The clinic was operating even more slowly than usual today and Martin was unusually irritated at the waste of time. His mother chided him gently on his impatience and he instantly felt remorseful. It was so hard to keep his different lives in perspective. Everything in her life had to go slowly. It must irk her that others could rush about and complete tasks efficiently and smoothly and without pain. These regular check ups for her severe arthritis were important to his mother, disabled as she was by this cruel affliction. It wasn't her fault that Melanie had got right under his skin and disturbed his usual calm.

Martin had always enjoyed a very close relationship with his mother. She was so accepting. He had never heard her rail against a fate that had rendered her so twisted and made her endure so much suffering. He knew when it was really bad because she became so quiet, as if it was too much effort even to speak. But on good days her lively humour and sheer enjoyment of life inspired him. Her brain was so agile that he sometimes wondered if it had overcompensated for the body's deficiencies. Many a long evening he enjoyed, stimulated by the cut and thrust of debate of some contentious issue and marvelled at how well read she had remained. The only problem was she knew him rather too well for his own comfort. It was nearly impossible to hide from her when he was disturbed by happenings at the hospital. And he always felt his appeal to patients' rights to confidentiality sounded rather lame.

He had grown even closer to her when his own life had been shattered by tragedy. The clinic chair was hard, unyielding. The waiting seemed endless. His eyes wandered to the poster exhorting him to consult the doctor if he suffered from a range of symptoms - made him feel ill just reading them. He focused on the damp spot above the door marked 'No entry except to authorised persons'. No threat there. Undemanding - a damp patch. He was back to that day five years ago. The young policeman had been so ill at ease. But how did they train these youngsters? How did they learn how to tell you your wife had been killed suddenly in a road accident. Martin felt again the unreality - then the utter devastation. How could you possibly accept the sudden extinction of a beautiful flame haired girl of 26, with a joy of life that challenged her to live it to the full?

He remembered all those fearful farewells as she set off for some daring adventure - sky diving - mountain walking - stock car racing. She had always departed in a whirl of embraces, shouted messages and false starts. For him there had only been the uneasy silence that descended on their tiny flat. She was so vivacious - so full of exuberant high spirits. Her going always left such a vacuum. What had she seen in him - a rather staid, mousey kind of a chap, fonder of books and quiet country walks than of anything remotely dangerous. And yet they had been supremely happy together, each free to pursue their own inclinations, secure in the certain knowledge that the other would be there for them at the end of the day.

Ironic that her death had not been during one of her madcap excursions. No, it was a very ordinary Wednesday morning. Vivienne had been off to see their GP. Thought she was pregnant - well, she was sure as she could be. Best get it confirmed - make it official, she'd said. They were so thrilled. First baby. First of lots he'd hoped. He was on tenterhooks all morning waiting for her to ring - tell him it was real - he was going to be a Dad. He'd call at the florist's on his way home - get her her favourite freesias - liked them better than red roses she always maintained. Every special date he bought her freesias. This was specially special - maybe chocolates too.

When the policeman came he hadn't been able to readjust. Too big a leap from being almost a Dad - waiting for the confirmation - the confirmation that never came. Not almost a Dad - a widower. A childless widower. How old and grey it sounded. He forced himself to listen. The words were halting, pained - poor young man struggling to articulate the unthinkable. Fidgeting with his helmet; not daring to look him in the eye. The bus driver maintained Viv had seemed in a bit of a dream - just stepped off the pavement in front of him. Nothing he could do to stop from hitting her at full speed. Two lives wiped out in one cruel moment. Was she so excited thinking about the baby that she hadn't looked where she was going? He knew now she had had the pregnancy confirmed - the GP told him afterwards she'd been so pleased she'd kissed him. Most unlike her. And now he was hearing this stranger telling him Viv was dead. Killed outright. And the baby dead too. Two lives wiped out in a second of time. Infinity left to mourn.

Identifying Viv had been worse than any nightmare. The double decker had done its worst. Nothing would ever erase that sight from his memory and the sick horror would always return to haunt him. He remembered all those weeks locked in a silent cocoon - every other living soul debarred. Only the aching, despairing grief - the emptyness.

It had been his mother who eventually reached in to him and drew him slowly back into life - a very different world now. He knew that a certain part of him would never heal. But she had oh so gently helped him to see that his self pity was not the finest tribute he could pay to Viv. He had to reconstruct his life - make her memory live on in some way. He felt, without any sense of self congratulation, that it did. It was the enormity of his own experience that had made him feel the pain of other wounded souls. A more acute sensitivity guided him now in his pastoral work. Not for him contented platitudes. He was not afraid of those bitter tears. He understood - really felt - the anguish that evoked the angry diatribes and hurled the potted plant at the glass door.

Her gentle sensivitity throughout those bitter years had made his mother someone very special to Martin. She had never once told him she knew how he felt. He so much appreciated that. It was such a different thing to lose a spouse naturally from illness at a good old age. How could that compare with the trauma of his loss of a young wife and a baby? Even as time passed and he recognized the common elements in loss - ceased to think of himself as uniquely singled out for suffering; he valued his mother's willingness to listen to his story without overlaying her own. There was real regret that he had not been more understanding of her grief when his father had died, so immersed was he in his own loss of the man who had always been such a special part of his life. But she had dismissed his apology, assuring him that he had helped - just being there - sorrowing too.

At first - after Viv - his mother had insisted that he move in with her, so she could 'look after him'. But he needed his privacy too much to sacrifice the flat and move into her more spacious home on a more permanent basis. They both knew it wouldn't work. They would irritate each other at too close quarters. So they developed an easy habit of phoning often. He dropped by frequently - ferried her around as she wished. But when he needed solitude he could escape to the home he had built up with his golden girl - brood, meditate, weep - without his mother feeling her overwhelming urge to make things better. She, too, could close the door secure in the knowledge that furniture she had so painfully polished would remain in position, free from coffee cups. Towels, chairs, coats, baskets - everything would remain neatly in place. No more stooping so agonisingly low to retrieve the dropped newspaper. Over the years a comfortable mutual acceptance had developed. They were both content with the arrangement.

Her time with the registrar today was if anything even briefer than it customarily was. For the umpteenth time, Mrs Lakes answered the usual questions about her drugs, her exercises, her mobility. The cheery injunction to keep up the good work rather grated on her as she looked at the young woman's flexible limbs and brisk movements. She sighed inwardly. Was it worth all the effort of coming just for such a cursory check? And just what was she thanking this young woman for? Had she in fact done anything? Oh well, it seemed the right thing to do.

The journey home was delayed by roadworks in the High Street and it was 3.35pm when Martin arrived back at the hospital. A message was waiting for him. Would he go up to the Special Care nursery for a christening. He groaned aloud. After the events of the day so far this was all he didn't need.

These were the worst calls he ever got - going to see these babies people thought were dying. It wasn't only his own sense of impotence in the face of the overwhelming grief of the parents. It wasn't just the look and the feel of those scrawny creatures with such a flickering hold on life. Nor was it really the way the staff wanted to unburden their sorrow too. Of course, all these factors impinged on his feelings too, but it was of his own loss that he couldn't help but think first. There had been no farewell for his baby. No-one else to say they were sorry. No-one else knew. It had been his and Viv's secret; shared on that fateful Wednesday with the doctor. Not even his mother knew. And he'd never been able to tell her since. It seemed somehow too precious and too sacred a secret to share with anyone but Viv; too painful a bereavement to add the loss of a grandchild to that of a daughter-in-law.

Collecting the tools of his trade, Martin took the lift to the Nursery. When he put his head round the office door, Sister Catherine Woollard was engrossed in papers which looked very like the duty rosters. At his tap, she raised her eyes and he was warmed by her instant smile.

'Oh thanks for coming, Martin. This is a difficult one, I'm afraid. Mum is a single girl and she is at loggerheads with her parents, especially her mother. Father of the baby scarpered when he found out about the pregnancy. It's Granny who wants Crystal baptised.'

'Crystal?' Martin rolled his eyes in exaggerated horror and Catherine laughed.

'Crystal Samantha Kimberley as I live and breathe!'

'So is Mum going to be present?'

'Yes, she says she's not going to leave her mother opportunities to do things for her grandchild without her say so. So she is there to make sure only the bare minimum to save Crystal's soul is permitted!'

'Makes it all into superstitious claptrap, doesn't it?' Martin replied with an ironic lift of one eyebrow.

Catherine grinned her agreement but both knew that they were required to go along with such requests no matter what their own views.

'Were you waiting long for me for this one?' Martin asked.

'No, not long. Why? Been busy?'

'Got stuck in the traffic in the High Street and was delayed getting back from another appointment so I didn't know when your message had come through,' Martin explained.

Catherine accompanied the chaplain to the nursery where Crystal Samantha Kimberley fought for every breath. Martin bit his lip at the purpleness of her skin and the wizened features pursed around the tube connecting her body to the huge ventilator. She scarcely looked human, he thought. She reminded him of fledgling birds he's seen in his youth, splattered on the path, ejected from faraway nests - so fragile he was always afraid to pick them up lest they were crushed by his touch. What would his baby have looked like if this was the result of 24 weeks incubation in a mother's womb? Instantly he forced the thought away and turned to the nurse who was looking after Crystal.

'OK if I just open the portholes and hold her head as I sprinkle her?' he enquired.

'Yes, you can't do much harm here now.'

Martin draped his stole around his neck and arranged the crisp white cloth and clear glass font on the trolley beside the incubator as Catherine left them to go to the family room to summon the mother and grandmother. Today it was too painful to stand there gazing at this blighted being. So he wandered over to the window and stood struggling to compose himself for what the next few minutes would entail. He turned at the sound of the door opening and there was no hint of his own internal turmoil as he smiled kindly at the young girl approaching him. She looked as if she should have been behind a desk learning arithmetic rather than haunting the corridors of death. Her eyes were red and swollen from crying and she clutched a sodden tissue and a brand new teddy bear in one fist as she walked towards the incubator. Catherine introduced her as Crystal's Mum and fresh tears welled as she laid a limp dampness in the chaplain's outstretched hand.

Behind the young mother came her parents. The grandmother had a grim tightness about her mouth which, with her severely scraped back greasy hair, gave her an austerity which was at odds with the poignancy of this moment, Martin felt. The grandfather was very tall and rather cumbersomely overweight. He portrayed an affable scruffiness which seemed to defy anyone to take this whole thing too seriously.

The motley group stood awkwardly, for a moment no-one quite sure what etiquette the bizarre circumstances of this ceremony demanded. Catherine broke the uneasy silence by putting an arm around the waist of the young mother and gently shepherding her to the far side of the incubator.

'Do you feel like holding Crystal's hand while Mr Lakes christens her?' she asked gently. A tearful shake of the untidy head loosened more tears. They dripped on to the dusky maroon floor turning into blood red splashes as they fell.

'OK.' Catherine's instant acceptance of her decision was soothing. 'Then how about if you stand here and then you can see everything easily.' She guided the girl to a position as near as she could stand to the baby's head. Returning to the other side she indicated the opposite end for the girl's parents leaving space for Martin to carry out his offices.

It was all over in a few moments and Martin was glad of the set rituals which enabled him to hold himself distant from the intimacy of the family's pain whilst preserving the solemnity of this act. But all too soon it was necessary for the elusive words of comfort. Did such words exist? By this time both mother and grandmother were in tears, thrown together by the shared acknowledgement that time was running out for Crystal. The sound of their sobbing contrasted strangely with the rhythmic whooshing of the ventilator maintaining this charade of breathing. He felt perversely relieved when, ignoring him, they left the room precipitately. The grandfather, less agile in his obesity and perhaps reluctant to re-enter their distress, lingered, staring down at his granddaughter with an expression of total incomprehension on his rather coarse features.

'Och, Meenister, - it's got me beat. Puir wee thing. Sae perfick whin they're sae wee,' he breathed. 'It's fair amazin', like.'

Martin, instantly recognizing the bewilderment of this man who had never seen a premature infant before, moved a fraction nearer.

'Yes, each little part so perfectly formed. It's all very wonderful but hard to understand all the same.'

'It is that. Wunnerfu'. D'ye think she's - ken - sufferin'?'

Catherine Woollard who had stepped back respectfully for the christening now came forward and in answer to Martin's raised eyebrows, replied, 'No, we don't think she is, Mr Caitland. We've given her something to keep her comfy.'

'How much - ken - longer, d'ye think?'

'Very difficult to say, I'm afraid. But it's likely to be today sometime we think,' the sister's voice was very soft and the hushed tones in which they all spoke preserved the dignity of these last few hours of the short life of a human being who would never really be known.

'M'lassie - she'll tak' it bad. She wus ne'er guid - ken - wi' deyin'. Grat buckets whin th' goldfish deid. An' whin th' hamster went, she kep' diggin' it up - checkin' it wus reelly deid. Couldnae dae nothin' wi' 'er - no' fur weeks.'

'It's very hard to go through something like this.' Martin said. 'And she's very young for such a hard experience.'

'Aye. Ye're richt ther. An' she an' the missus - they dinnae git on noo. Fight like cat an' dug. Since she foond oot - ken - 'boot the bairn. Bu' mebees things'll git better - ken - aifter like.' His hopeful sentiment was belied by his lugubrious expression as he shook his head over Crystal. Abruptly he straightened his shoulders and turning to Martin, said 'Thanks, Meenister, Ah'm fair gratefu'. Th' missus, wud thank ye an' a' - and th' wean - but they cannae stop greetin'.'

'Don't mention it. I shall be thinking of you all and please if you think it would help, do send for me. I'm most willing to help but I don't want to intrude.' Martin warmly grasped the big man's hand in both his own. With a nod he ambled out.

Catherine waited just long enough to thank Martin and tell him she must go and see the mother was all right. However, just as she was leaving the nursery she turned back and asked, 'I was wondering - are you around this evening? There's something - I'd like to talk to you - if you have the time.'

Martin was conscious of a devout wish to go home and simply fold up. People didn't seem to understand that he wasn't an automaton or a bottomless jug of compassion. He too had his limits and his breaking points. But who knew about those? No-one, he suspected. Ah well at least there was no-one at home to complain that he never kept to time and was never in and when he did come home he was too exhausted for civilised conversation. A great surge of sadness enveloped him. He was having a maudlin sort of a day, he reflected - must try to snap out of it. Nothing of his struggle showed as he gave his customary response.

'I can be, certainly. What kind of time were you thinking of?'

'When I finish this evening about 9.30ish? Or is that too late?'

'No, that's fine. I'll be in my office downstairs. If I'm called out I'll leave a message for you.'

'Thanks a lot.' Catherine hurried off in pursuit of the distressed relatives, grateful for this gentle man's presence.

Peace again descended on the little group in the nursery. Unhurriedly Martin packed away his equipment, quietly conversing with the remaining nurse, Jane Featherstone, as she attended to Crystal's mouth. It pleased him that the staff accepted his presence so easily that they continued with their routine work even while he remained in the nursery once his official function was completed.

'Tough on you, too, watching her go,' he said.

'Yes, it's not nice. But at least we haven't had this one for months. You don't know them like little people in their own right then. When we've had them for ages they become real little characters and it breaks your heart then. I cry with the parents sometimes.'

'I'm sure that's a great comfort to them. It must help to know that the staff cared enough to grieve too. And at least it's not frowned on - not like it used to be - showing your own emotion I mean.'

'Oh I know - went out with the starched aprons I guess!' They both laughed. 'But it's an odd thing, you know.' Jane's brow puckered as she spoke. 'Even though, umm, you don't want them to linger and, ah, you honestly think it's best - best that they die quickly, I mean - you still hope - hope that it won't be while you're looking after them.'

'Uhhmmm.' Martin's nod encouraged her to pursue the point.

'It's not just, umm, that you don't want to deal with the rellies or do the last offices or anything. But sometimes it feels like you haven't done your job very well - if you let one of them die, I mean. I can't explain it, but, umm, well that's how I feel. But if they die when someone else is in charge of them, I never think, 'Oh she didn't do very well' - it's only when it's me.'

'Mmmm, that's interesting but I think I know what you mean. We have such mixed-up feelings - about death, don't we?' She flashed him a grateful smile for his ready understanding. 'Look, I'm a bit out on a limb when it comes to death actually. So don't quote me on this one.' Martin drew a little nearer as he confided his hitherto unspoken opinion. 'I'm a layman. I'm not a doctor. But I really do feel that perhaps part of our problem is - well, we find it so hard to accept death as natural - a natural part of life. We sort of feel we have to fight it - tooth and nail. Feels like a failure when someone does die. We've let them down. I think it was Illich who called death the ultimate form of consumer resistance, wasn't it?' They both grinned at the analogy.

'There's this sort of sense that we just can't let the enemy win! But I feel that p'rhaps if we saw death, not as a scientific failure, but as the inevitable endpoint of medical and nursing care - and if everything was moving towards that point - we'd feel very differently about it. D'you see what I mean? I'm not expressing it very well. But that's my feeling anyway.'

'I think I understand. But I'd need to think about it.'

'It wouldn't then be a question of: We must try everything aggressively to prevent this person dying - to stop us failing. It would be more: OK this person's going to die - whatever we do. Is it sensible to delay that process? Now you'll probably shoot me down in flames!' Martin looked rather shyly at Jane giving a self-deprecating shake of his head as he spoke.

Jane continued sucking out Crystal's secretions thankful for the pause for reflection the noisy suction machine gave her. Then as she disposed of the catheter and settled the baby on her tummy, she responded slowly.

'No, I think I see your point. I'd need to think it through more - before I could agree or disagree. But it's interesting - different. And it could explain, umm, why I feel so badly if they die when I'm in charge of them. It could make life a whole lot easier - if you didn't see it as a failure, I mean - blame yourself. Like you say. But, I'll need to think some more on that.'

Martin realized his conclusion had been a long time coming to him even though he had pondered these things for many years. He decided to leave it at that and with a smile, bade Jane goodbye before returning to his office to collect papers for a seminar he was leading for first-year medical students. He thoroughly enjoyed these sessions. Didactic lecturing he found tedious; bored with his own material after so many repetitions. But he loved the challenge of interactive work. The refreshing views of these new recruits appealed to him, and he took real pleasure in offering them an extension of their thinking or a diametrically opposed argument and watching them grappling with the ramifications and consequences. Today's session was on abortion and he hoped there would be some radical thinkers to stimulate everyone into lively discussion. His fellow presenter was Dr Tony Croft, a gynaecologist with some interesting ideas of his own, who was sufficiently confident and experienced to present whichever view would best encourage analytical thinking. It promised to be a good hour.

It was not until eight o'clock that evening that Martin had the luxury of a few moments respite to acknowledge his tiredness. The teaching session had been one of the best ones so far with powerful arguments being sharpened on both sides of the abortion debate. The buzz had remained with him for the next couple of hours as he popped back to see Melanie - only to find her deeply asleep - and then kept an appointment with an overseas medical student who was having housing problems. Sorry as he was for the Nigerian, he could deal with such practical matters without having to engage his feelings and he welcomed the necessity to concentrate on this man's difficulties blotting out the emotional drains of the earlier hours. He now had an hour and a half to catch up with paper work before the Sister from the Neonatal Unit arrived. He wondered rather idly what she wanted to talk about that was pressing enough and delicate enough to require a session at this hour away from the Unit. But no point in speculation - he'd soon know.

When the tap at his door roused him, he realized he had actually nodded off in mid-sentence of a report he was writing. He must have been more exhausted than he had thought. But the ten minutes nap would have refreshed him and he'd be able to keep going longer tonight. Catherine Woollard in her normal clothes looked so different from the senior figure of the Unit, he noted with some surprise. It flashed through his mind that it would be so easy to repeat the error of the nurse who, encountering an ex-patient in a shop, exclaims loudly, 'Oh, you look so different with your clothes on!' He stifled a grin and instead rose courteously to welcome her. As she accepted his offer of an orange juice he wondered if she was stalling for time, she seemed strangely ill at ease and vulnerable tonight. In her own domain, in the crisp but anonymous uniform, with always a specific purpose in mind, she seemed so self assured, so poised, so efficient and calm. Here in her jeans and a loose dusky pink sweater with her dark hair framing her small boned face instead of fastened high on her head, she looked defenceless, younger somehow, and rather shy. But he had been a chaplain for too many years to find small talk difficult so he set about putting her at ease with undemanding enquiries about the state of play in the Unit tonight, her plans for the new day-room and how she spent her leisure hours.

Catherine was indeed ill at ease. She had had a visit from Wendy - a very upset Wendy. Haltingly, over and over again saying she didn't want to cause any trouble, she had told her story. She was full of self-reproach. Had she got it badly wrong - in the Unit meeting? Jo Manson had been so angry. Was it her fault? It hadn't just been the meeting - Jo had rebuffed her efforts at peacemaking, afterwards in the changing room. Really hostile she was. Wendy sought reassurance. Had she been too dogmatic - too unkind? Wendy - unkind! What a nonsense it all was. But the girl was clearly deeply disturbed. Catherine took a long time, telling her repeatedly how good a neonatal nurse she was. How Jo seemed to have a chip on her shoulder. There were things in her past they didn't properly understand. But she'd been a prickly customer from the outset. No, it most definitely wasn't Wendy's fault. She had behaved calmly and reasonably. The aggression had all been on Jo's side. Even so, Catherine had felt a sinking feeling when Wendy had burst out with, 'It almost makes me want to go to the Pro-Life people. Just to get some reassurance!' It must be hard - feeling marginalized, holding an extreme viewpoint, a strong religious conviction. Catherine wished she could agree with Wendy - confirm her in her radical belief. Stop her taking this matter outside. But she couldn't. Her own beliefs, her experience - everything told her it just wasn't tenable. Not for her. She'd be lying to agree just for Wendy's short-term peace.

It had been so very unsatisfactory. She felt a great need to talk through her problem - with someone who was distant enough not to have their own relationships affected. But someone who knew the tensions, understood the issues. Martin had seemed like the answer when he'd been so kind with Crystal's family.

Now she felt the temerity of her request, keeping this man when he probably just wanted to get home. But he was being so friendly, so interested. Didn't seem like a chore. She began to relax.

The light from the anglepoise on the desk behind Catherine threw a halo round her head but left her face in shade. Martin had instinctively offered her this protection. She seemed to want to talk confidentially. He noted with some relief that she had stopped fidgetting.

'How may I help you?' he asked laying down his glass and folding his hands in his lap.

'Well, I wondered - if you wouldn't mind - if we could talk about the Unit meeting on Monday. You remember? The one about Peter Flanaghan?' He nodded. 'I mean, I don't mean I want to discuss Peter in particular ... Oh dear, I'm tying myself up in knots here.'

'It's OK. Take your time.'

'You know what I mean. I know you've done a lot of reading on the subject of decisions - about life and death. Well, what I really need - there are things I'd like to get clearer in my own mind.'

'OK, fire away.'

'Well, I don't know where to start really. I sort of have ideas but I can't give a rational explanation for why I think like I do. It's a sort of gut feeling. But I feel I ought to be able to back it up with something.'

'Uhhmmm. Don't be too hard on yourself - it's not so easy.'

'I suppose my worry is - well, it's really about what we're asking of the parents. I think perhaps it's not right to be asking them to decide whether their baby lives or dies. It's such a - such a - well - an awesome decision. And they have to live with it for the rest of their lives. Maybe we - you know, the staff - maybe we ought to make the decision. Be prepared for them to be angry with us. I feel it's probably better - easier - for them to be angry with us than with themselves. And maybe they **need** something - or somebody - to blame when things go so horribly wrong.'

Martin had been giving her his full attention and his periodic nods of understanding empowered her. She became more fluent as her reticence left her.

'I feel I'm being horribly old-fashioned about this - going back to the days where doctors were seen as all-powerful. Nobody dared question what they said, you know?'

'Paternalism rules. OK!' Martin grinned companionably at her, making a punching gesture into the air with his right clenched fist.

She smiled responsively.

'I **don't** think they know it all - the doctors. But on the other hand, if I'm flying to the States, I don't expect to tell the pilot how to fly the plane. When I take the car to the garage, I don't tell the mechanic how to do his job. So, why should parents expect to tell us how to look after their babies?' Martin opened his mouth to reply but she was in mid-thought.

'When I worked as a midwife in labour ward we got to a stage where women were coming in with a great list of things they wanted and I got really quite fed up at one point - they really didn't know what labour would be like but they'd heard or read various things were good or bad or whatever. I don't know, it feels as if they aren't trusting us - you know, to do our job well - to have their best interests at heart.'

'I understand what you're saying. But, I wonder - I just wonder, are these analogies quite fair? I'm thinking out loud now - haven't properly thought this through. It's difficult to find something that really equates to a human life, isn't it? I mean, if the car isn't right when it comes back from the garage, you can take it back and say, "Here you must fix this rattle or whatever." But when it's a child - it has to be a different kind of negotiation. You can't replace him. But OK, let's stick with your example and see where it takes us. P'rhaps it's a bit like having a car that's pretty much on its last legs and you take it to the garage and you say, "Fix this thing for me I need it to get to work every day and I have to go to Lands End next week." And the mechanic might look at it and fiddle about a bit and then say, "Well, you've got a choice here. I can fix the rattle - replace the carburretor - tighten up the exhaust" - or whatever they do - I don't know the first thing about how cars work! Don't know the big end from the dipstick!' The humour lightened Catherine's tension and she laughed with him.

'Nor me! So you can say what you like - I won't know any better.'

'OK. This mechanic - he says, "I can fix all these things and you can take it away. But," he says, "I can't guarantee it won't break down next time you're hurtling down the motorway. On the other hand", he says, "I could suggest that you trade it in for a newer model." And then it's up to you to decide what level of risk you're prepared to accept. If you're pretty good with tinkering with the engine yourself you might decide that, OK, it's worth hanging on to the clapped-out model - it's cheaper - and anyway you are quite attached to it. But if you're completely useless with engines you'll probably decide you need more security earlier. Unless you're a poor chaplain in which case you probably couldn't afford to replace it no matter how last-legsy it gets! But you see where I'm going?'

Catherine nodded vigorously. 'Uhhuh.'

'So is it telling someone how to do their job? Not exactly, I don't think. More like the expert - the mechanic, the doctor - giving the "owner" the facts - leaving them to decide how much of a risk they're prepared to take? Then - to get back to the babies - one family might decide they desperately want this baby at all costs. So even when the doctor says, "He's got a one in a 100 chance," they'll take it. But another family'll reason, "If we take this baby home with all those problems, severely handicapped and all that - it'll be the end of our marriage, our relationship with our other children, the end of our peace of mind, our sanity. We're not prepared to take that kind of gamble. We'll stick with what we've got. And anyway, OK he'd probably die in a few years anyway. We won't pull out all the stops - don't want to prolong such a miserable existence. We'll let him go now while we've still got good memories. While we can feel sad at losing him - not just relieved he's gone." Either way they're dependent on the expert, aren't they? - the doctor - for guidance. But they're the ones in the driving seat dealing with the consequences of the decision.'

'Yes, I see what you mean. And of course, they're the ones who have to live with whatever's decided. We move on to other cases and have all our other interests and activities to keep things in perspective. But they - they can never escape - from the consequence of the decision, I mean - whichever way it goes.'

'Absolutely. Whichever way it goes. It's an on-going sorrow to have a severely handicapped child. But it can also be an on-going sorrow to have agreed to a child dying, I'm convinced of that.'

'Oh I agree. I don't know how they cope, really. It's hard enough for us - and they're not our babies. We grieve too when they die. But it can't be as bad - not as bad as how the mothers feel. My worry is that they would also feel guilty - because they'd helped to make the decision - you know, that it was better for their baby not to exist than to continue even a painful or handicapped life.'

'Yes, I appreciate your worry. But my experience is that - they're helped to the decision very carefully. Dr Carshalton, I know, always tells them that he's responsible for the final decision. He encourages them to discuss the issues - how they feel. But he always says that they mustn't feel they're in anyway to blame for what happens. He's the one who'll stop the treatment, disconnect the tubes, and I'm sure you've seen the way he offers them the chance to hold the baby without all the tubes and things attached. He always says - it's really nice - he says they have a very special role to play in this last bit - it's a very special role - something nobody else can do. I specially like the way he emphasizes that the baby knows they're different - they're his parents - they're not the people who're always doing beastly things to him like sticking needles in, banging his chest about and everything. Their touch is different - all of that - it's lovely the way he makes them feel so special.'

Catherine was nodding, remembering with him so many vigils with dying infants and Roger Carshalton's special sensitivity with the parents.

'I think we're probably particularly lucky here with our consultants. They're so gentle - take time explaining things over and over again to the parents. But you could well imagine - you know, if you had someone who wasn't as sensitive steaming in - doing their own thing - and the parents getting a distinct impression that their baby was a bit of disposable flotsam to be discarded when a better candidate came in needing the incubator. Then I guess we'd be glad that there was a system of involving the parents.'

'Yes, I suppose if you've got good doctors it probably isn't too important - not so important anyway - just how much the parents are involved in the actual decision. So long as they're fully informed.' Catherine was looking deep into her glass totally absorbed in her musings.

'And then, of course,' Martin pursued his train of thought, 'It's only the parents who really know their circumstances, what resources they can muster and so on. So no-one else can really dictate how much of a burden they should shoulder.'

'I was interested in your comment at Monday's meeting - you know - when you asked about the value of the handicapped baby's life. If you think all life is of equal value, how does this quality of life - from the parents' point of view - fit in?' Catherine was looking directly at him now with her head slightly tilted in enquiry.

'In my own defence, I have to say, I don't think I stated my position at that meeting. You can be forgiven for thinking I did - people often jump to that conclusion! But I was actually just raising the point.' Martin smiled reassuringly. He wasn't in the least prickly about such misinterpretations.

'I raised it because I don't think we should ignore it. But if I could state my own personal point of view ...?'

'Please do. I'm interested.'

'Personally I draw my line between those who're physically and mentally handicapped. If they're just mentally handicapped then you can't withdraw treatment and allow them to die because they don't need treatment in the first place. And I'm definitely not into starving babies to death! If they're physically impaired then I think it's a matter of balancing burdens and benefits from the child's point of view. What seems more compassionate - to allow suffering so that the child lives, or to allow death as preferably to years of pain and distress? I suspect the line'll be drawn at a different point with each of us. But as long as we're only talking about the child's interests we are on the right lines. If you start to introduce the family's interests or society's or resource implications then, I think, you're on dangerous ground.'

'Now I'm confused! I thought we'd just said the family's perspective is important?'

'Yes, we did and it is. But when it comes to deciding about treatment withdrawal or continuance, then our first and primary consideration has to be the infant. What is in his best interests? Yes?' She nodded. 'When you're looking at the wider burdens and benefits you put everything else into the balance too - the family's feelings, resources, coping ability and so on. So I don't personally think it is ever right to allow a baby to die simply because the family don't want him.'

'Ah dear, it is complicated!' Catherine sighed. 'When I sit here listening to you it all seems so clear. But I can't seem to keep it all sorted in my own mind - I can't stick to a consistent argument when I'm in a spot. It all gets so muddled. You seem to be able to put it all in such an orderly and understandable way. I can't.'

'Well, if I can - and it's kind of you to say so - it's only because it's a special interest of mine and I've heard the points rehearsed so many times now. But I agree, these things are difficult to stay with somehow. You can easily lose the thread of what you're trying to say because there are so many tangents that are equally relevant and so many qualifying conditions that make loopholes where you really want absolutes. There's a lot of greyness about these things and we're more comfortable with black and white for the most part. Most people find philosophers hard to follow.'

'Well, that's reassuring.'

'But I'm no philosopher. I'm just a plain man looking at philosophical issues so I reinterpret the principles into real life situations, and then I feel I can start to get a handle on what we're talking about. But for someone like me there's always a danger that my limited experience will take me down a narrow track and there will be other examples from real life where what I've concluded just doesn't fit. Then I come back to the basic principles again. Oh dear! I sound like I'm sermonizing - sorry!'

'No, you're not at all.' Catherine dismissed the suggestion with a gesture of her hand.

'Don't be too hard on yourself.' Martin advised. 'You're probably better to concentrate on being sure of your own position and that it holds water and not worry too much about being able to justify it with a nice series of logical arguments! You're in a much stronger position than me - you've got so much experience of these babies under your belt. I suspect that mostly people will listen to what you say and not need lengthy explanation. You know because you've been there and done that. I know I'm very often persuaded by people like yourself who have actually **lived** these experiences.'

'Well, that's encouraging to hear. But even so, I feel pretty inadequate to myself. If, for example, someone said, 'Well, I don't think quality of life issues come into it, it's a more fundamental matter of the sanctity of life itself,' I'd be flummoxed. I sort of know that pain and suffering are relevant but I'd be hard put to it to say why. I don't want to suffer so why should I decide that **others** must. I guess that's about it.'

Catherine was wanting so much to confide in him about her particular concerns at this precise time. All the anxiety Wendy and Jo had created preyed on her mind. Was she equal to the task of steering a course through this minefield without casualties. But loyalty and a deep respect for confidences restrained her and she kept to generalities.

'Absolutely, and that's exactly right. It's one of the two well-established moral ideals - treat others as you would wish them to treat you. The old 'Golden rule', as it's called.'

'And what's the other one?'

'That we ought to do our best to relieve or avoid unnecessary suffering. That gives us a responsibility in medicine to consider what our treatments mean in terms of suffering - and whether the prospect for the future merits inflicting pain or injury or whatever. I'm sure you've looked at some patients with advanced cancer and wondered why someone decrees that they should spend their last weeks vomiting their hearts up, constantly nauseated and off their food, hairless and so on and so on as a result of chemotherapy. What's it all for? I know I have.'

Catherine was nodding vigorously. Martin was enjoying this discussion with someone who was clearly so interested in the issues which exercised his mind so often. He continued, hoping that he wasn't being too 'preachy'. His mother sometimes told him he sounded like a minister when he was talking with her.

'And I also know I personally wouldn't want to forgo some degree of dignity in such a hopeless situation - well, I only mean hopeless in the sense of medically futile. I think then we need to change the direction we're looking in - see the death as the inevitable endpoint and decide how we reach it with the minimum of discomfort and distress and the maximum of dignity, peace of mind and comfort. Whoops, sermon again! Sorry! But it's an interesting paradox that physicians who've been surveyed would want to stop treatment for themselves far sooner than they're prepared to stop it for their patients. I think that speaks volumes.'

Catherine laughed with him. 'Interesting! But you've just demonstrated what I'm concerned about. You have it all neatly summarized in two - what did you call them - moral what?'

'Moral ideals.'

'OK, two moral ideals. Then it all sounds so - I don't know, creditable, legit, acceptable. But I wouldn't know to sum it up so succinctly. By the time I've rephrased it in pidgin English, it sounds so puny.'

'You're underestimating your powers of persuasion. There was a fascinating debate between Ian Kennedy - you know who I mean? One of **the** leading exponents in these matters with a legal mind you have to admire.' Catherine was nodding. 'Well, he was debating with a group of medical men and afterwards someone summed it up rather neatly. They said Ian Kennedy knocked the spots off the doctors who just couldn't compete with the cleverness of his words and the masterly command of the arguments he could demonstrate. He made them look and feel foolish. But, the commentator said, if I was ill and needed attention I'd far rather have any one of those doctors to care for me than Ian Kennedy! They knew first-hand about compassion and caring. So take heart! Go with those gut feelings born of so many deeply moving experiences. I think your heart will keep you right even if your brain and tongue don't quite keep up with it!'

'You are kind. And I do feel better for having talked to you. It's been bugging me for ages and that meeting on Monday brought it all to the surface. I was almost afraid to open my mouth for fear of sounding so pathetic. And here I am in charge of the Unit! And I must admit - but this is in confidence - things are still a bit rocky in some quarters as a result of that meeting and what it revealed about certain individuals. But I know you've studied these things so I thought - I hoped - you wouldn't mind if I had a chat tonight.'

'I don't mind at all. In fact I've enjoyed chatting to you - in the Unit we always seem to just concentrate on the work. It's good to get away from that atmosphere and talk in a more relaxed way - get to know one another better.'

'I've enjoyed it too. Thanks very much.'

'I don't know how much further you want to take this but if you're keen to get it sorted out - just for your own peace of mind - you might find it helpful to make a sort of summary of the arguments on both sides - in your own words - a sort of list that means something to you - a ready reference.' Martin's suggestion was offered tentatively. He was anxious not to be pushing her into a deeper level of thinking if that wasn't what she was seeking.

'Yes, that would be good. I'm not quite sure how I'd go about it. Unless ... could you - would you mind - giving me some references - just to get me started, do you think, please? No hurry, of course. Just when you find a spare minute and if you wouldn't mind.' Was she asking too much? Catherine bent over backwards to give him an escape route.

'I'd be happy to.' His instant response warmed her and she visibly relaxed her shoulders. 'In fact I'll lend you a couple of books right now to get you going - if you'd like?' His tone and lifted eyebrow gave her permission to decline if she wished to. But she was grateful for his help.

'That would be great, thanks a lot.'

Martin rose at once and selected two fairly slim volumes from his large collection of books.

'Let me know how you fare with those and if you want more let me know.' He placed them almost nonchalantly on the table beside her not wishing to hand them directly to her in case she felt he was too insistent on her taking them.

Catherine picked them up at once conscious of the lateness of the hour and rose to her feet rather suddenly. Gathering up her abandoned jacket she slipped it on, flicking her swathe of dark hair from under the collar, with a practised hand, so that it cascaded on to her shoulders. Martin briefly thought how much prettier she looked stripped of the trappings of authority.

He cut her thanks short saying sincerely, 'Really, I've enjoyed it. There aren't too many people who enjoy considering these philosophical points and it's been good to discuss them with someone who's genuinely interested instead of the people who must endure my ramblings!'

'Thanks again. I'll take good care of your books and get them back to you as soon as I can.' Her smile gave him a warm feeling. The thought of his solitary flat held little appeal. A sudden impulse made him act quite uncharacteristically.

'It's been a long day - I'm starving. Have you eaten? I don't suppose - would you be interested - perhaps a pizza?'

'That would be lovely - yes, I'm ravenous. Why don't we.'

'I sometimes go to that little place on Montgomery Street. But I hate eating alone. You'd be doing me a great favour.'

He packed up his papers, rinsed the two glasses and locked the office door without a backward glance.

CHAPTER 7

Medical Musings

Roger walked briskly along the corridor. In the two days since the Unit meeting to discuss Peter Flanaghan's destiny he had given a great deal of thought to how best to elicit the honest feelings of his medical colleagues. Scarcely noticing the familiar signposts to wards and departments in this vast warren of a hospital, his mind went back to that evening with Tom Faithful.

Strange fellow - likeable enough if you weren't put off by that rough exterior. He'd been through the mill - infertility - marriage breaking up. Seemed lonely. But he was a good clinician - at least he was good with the babies. Pity about the way he dealt with the nurses. A lot of tension around there.

He didn't seem to have very strong opinions either way when it came to the life and death stuff. But, in Peter's case, he seemed to favour stopping treatment sooner rather than later. Roger was slightly disconcerted by Tom's essentially pragmatic approach. He had been patently uninterested in the moral reasoning - hadn't risen to any of the baits Roger had thrown out. OK he'd said he had no religious scruples - honest about that anyway. Being so direct helped. But you'd have thought his clinical experience might have given him a view. Four years in neonatology must have shown him that babies and families didn't follow the guidebook. What was right in one case might well not be in another. In fairness he did have a view - it was just rather general - not very deep. He tended to want to spare the babies suffering.

Roger felt rather envious of Tom's apparently casual attitude to death. He got a distinct impression that flicking the switch that turned off the ventilator would be rather like shutting the porthole of the incubator to Dr Faithful. Not a matter to lose sleep over. But he might be quite mistaken - underneath that unmoved exterior there might well be deep feelings ruthlessly suppressed. He'd had a lot of practice suppressing feelings, Tom.

Ira Ramshanshani - now she was an altogether different kettle of fish. Superb house officer. Cut above the usual calibre. Came with a glittering list of distinctions. Girl with a great future ahead. But better still - modest, warm, friendly with it. Winning combination. Hadn't allowed her academic successes to give her an inflated opinion of herself - not like some of the brightest students. No, Ira undertook even the most menial and tedious tasks with charm and good humour. He appreciated that. And she'd shown herself tough enough to cope with the sleepless nights - all those crises which bombarded the tired brain at 3am as relentlessly as they did at civilised hours. He'd like to see her continue in neonatology. She'd make a good colleague.

Stephen McDonald, the other house officer, was much less aspiring - much less inspired too come to think of it. Came from the same year as Ira at medical school. Hearty sort of fellow. Quite happy to scrape by on the minimum of work. He did his job - just. But he seemed much more interested in getting off for golf and playing with his computer - obsessive about that computer he was. Roger had felt quite exasperated by his excuses about late arrivals to take over the shift from Ira - had to finish some programme or other. Didn't seem to think about her needs. And she looked so drained sometimes at the end of a long and difficult session on duty. Odd how some of these chaps could be so blind. Made you wonder what kind of doctors they'd become. So much of it was observation.

When Roger had asked him how he felt about the Flanaghan's situation he'd been so offhand. Might have been deciding which club to use for the next shot. Seemed not to be considering the seriousness of it all. Quite happy just to leave it to those who knew - those were his words. Knew what? Didn't he realize he wouldn't be able to hide behind others all his life? Roger felt a distinct sense of relief that Stephen would be moving on in three months time. Not the sort of fellow you wanted around distraught parents.

He arrived at the door to the Neonatal Unit almost without realizing it. For the next hour and a half all thoughts of the debate about Peter were obliterated by the need to concentrate on each baby in his care. The discussion with the rest of the team was, as ever, brisk and helpful. Plenty of interesting cases to show to the students. They left Peter till last. As he stood looking down at the worn old-man face, lips pursed around his endotracheal tube, all the heartache flooded back. Resist it as he might, he couldn't stop himself from taking it all rather personally. He so much wanted to reassure Sue and Richard that all would be well - it was just a question of being patient. He hated to lose these little creatures. Especially the ones they'd fought so hard for. Felt like a blot on the copybook. Silly really. You couldn't save them all. No-one could. But he still hated it.

The satellite staff and medical students dispersed. Ira smiled as she slid the last folder of notes into its file, clipping her pen into the top pocket of her white coat.

'Coffee?' she enquired.

'Love one,' Roger responded instantly. 'Could we take it along to the Quiet Room? I'm still bothered about the Flanaghan family? I'd welcome a chance to talk it through a bit. Have you got time just now?'

Ira was always warmed by Roger's approach. She had worked for chiefs who ordered rather than asked and she appreciated his tacit acknowledgement that she had her commitments and timetable too. She agreed readily and led the way to the staff room where the fragrance of coffee beckoned. They chatted idly about the weather and their plans for the coming weekend as they poured drinks and walked along the corridor to the room reserved for telling bad news or having quiet talks with relatives.

It was a softly furnished room, the homely touches Catherine Woollard had added making it into an approachable environment. The parents, lost and bewildered by this alien place, needed such a sanctuary. How many times Roger had sat in those beige chairs explaining the complicated medical facts about their baby to dazed and shocked families. Mothers, fathers, grandmothers, grandfathers - they'd all sat here - cradling their dying infants in the muted peace of this withdrawn place, clutching like drowning men at each moment of loving. This was a space which tried to soften the edges of cruelty. A room for letting go.

Aware that their peace might be shattered at any moment Roger launched straight into his subject.

'Can I ask you - how do you feel about Peter's continuing treatment?'

'Me, personally?'

'Yes.'

'I wouldn't want to continue if he were mine. For them? More difficult. My sense of where these parents are at - is - is that they aren't yet ready to make this decision. So I'd want to keep going, if Peter can stand it, until they are ready.'

'OK. I know - from what you said at the Monday meeting - that you've broached the subject - tentatively - with the parents.'

'Uhhuh.'

'But I'm actually really wanting a feel for what you think yourself.'

'Fine.'

'Aside from the severe disability, the prospect is pretty bleak, as you know. We could give the little chap a trache, send him home with oxygen, keep plugging the antibiotics - and so on and so on. You know the name of the game with these chronic cases. But - I hope you don't mind my asking - how do you - you personally - feel about stopping now rather than going that far?'

'Well, I must admit, quality of life is something I personally feel pretty strongly about. I feel - this kind of scenario - it's appalling from the point of view of both Peter, and the parents. It's no life for him, poor litle soul - having all this painful treatment. But I guess - only the parents can decide really when the burdens outweigh the benefits - from the whole family's point of view. I'm not convinced - from what I've seen - that Sue is made of the stuff of saints. But I might be wrong. She could recover from this shock - go on to be much more robust than she is now. People do.'

'So, you wouldn't be averse to stopping treatment - now?' Roger was trying to be clear in his own mind where she stood.

'No....' The single syllable was drawn out as Ira thought through her response. 'I've been - giving this quite a bit of thought lately.' She bit her lip in concentration. 'I think I know where I stand myself. The bit that's bugging me is - the rights issue. I'm less clear about where people's rights begin and end. And one thing I definitely am confused about is whether people actually have a right to die. You know, babies can sue us for wrongful life; parents can sue us for negligence; we can be accused of attempted murder! But when it comes down to it - so much seems to hang on understanding the limits and boundaries. Does this kiddie - Peter - have a right to die? Does **anyone** have a right to die?'

'Good question. How long have you got for this one?' Roger laughed as he spoke, aware that time in the Unit was not their's to command. 'I find this whole thing complex - a bit eel-like.' She obviously didn't understand this reference. 'Just when you think you've grasped it, it slips away again. Eel-like.'

'Oh, I see!'

'And if you read the legal submissions from the test cases you end up rather more confused than you began. But I'll try to address it as I understand it - just don't quote me on this one!'

Ira smiled broadly and settled more comfortably to give him her full attention.

'It's awfully fashionable nowadays to talk about "rights",' Roger's fingers traced the apostrophes in the air. 'The right to procreate, the right to life; the right not to have been born; the right to clean air; the right to have sex with a person of the same gender; the right to streak naked across the Wimbledon courts! You know - we see it all.'

'Yes, I know what you mean.'

'But my feeling is that people tend to use "rights" to mean "wants" a lot of the time. Take the right to have a child. I don't know about you, but I don't personally think women do have an absolute right to procreate. There are other interests at stake than simply those of the woman. What are the child's rights? Where the mother is in a lesbian relationship? Where the parent smokes? Where they're drug addicts? Where the mother's 65?'

'Yes - it's highlighted with these much older mothers.'

'So I personally have a problem - with using the language of rights - when it comes to dying. It's hard enough - when you have to tackle these heart-rending cases like Peter Flanaghan - to work out what's morally right - what's in the best interests of the different individuals. Adding demands about a legal or moral 'right to die' complicates things still further. But then, perhaps that's because I find it difficult, logically, to defend any such thing as a "right to die".'

'These philosophical and moral arguments fascinate me but I'm not good at articulating them,' Ira broke in.

'I know exactly what you mean. Easy to get bogged down in all the complexities.'

'I'm with you so far on the problem of using the idea of rights to talk about dying.'

Her prompting encouraged Roger to pursue the topic in the same vein.

'I think actually this whole business is rather important. It reflects something of what our society holds dear. Our willingness to protect the vulnerable. It's not really about the articulate or the vocal minority fighting on issues like abortion or AIDS. They can defend themselves for the most part. It's about the weak and the defenceless ones who can't fight for themselves.' Roger's thoughts went, inevitably, to his daughter. Ira knew nothing of her, however, and neither saw anything to indicate this was anything more than a professional exchange.

'I take the point.'

'But you asked specifically about a supposed "right to die"? A "right" - to me - is not the same thing as a want or a desire. I might want to go to Tenerife for a holiday but I don't have an inalienable right to such a holiday! Nor is it - a capacity to have something. I have a capacity to take home the lab equipment for my personal use, but I don't have any right to do so!'

Ira was smiling broadly at his pertinent illustrations.

'So a "right", it seems to me, is rather a form of liberty. If it really is a "right" - a true "right" - it should in principle be absolute and unconditional. Something you can do without anyone else interfering or opposing it. Rights allow us to protect our own safety - our own dignity - against dictators - against high-minded moralisers. Yes?' She nodded again, this time less emphatically, not quite sure where this was going. Roger slowed the pace of his argument.

'But then for every right I have, someone else has some kind of obligation or responsibility. And there's one of the sticking points if we come back to this "right to die".'

Ira felt more secure. Some of the distinctions were confusing - this one she could grasp. She'd been there. Her mind raced back to an incident when she was doing her medical house job. Joseph Laird had been dying. No doubt about it. In his late 80s - oesophageal varices - he'd had three massive haemorrhages. Liver shot to pieces. Now he had a stubborn chest infection. The on-going anaemia had made him so weak. He was fighting for every breath - said it was agony to inhale. Even the continuous oxygen, the nebulizer - nothing made much difference. When he hadn't made it - didn't get the bedpan in time - that had tipped him over the edge. He'd pleaded - she could see his eyes yet - pleading - gripping her arm so hard it hurt. Give him something to end it all.

Until that precise moment, she'd been a textbook sympathiser. Yes, she believed in euthanasia - in principle. But she knew then - she knew when Joseph Laird clutched at her arm and her heartstrings - rights carried obligations. She couldn't do it. She felt sick. Oh she understood - understood very well what made him ask. She'd want it too in his circumstances. But you couldn't. It wasn't like a dog. She was a doctor. He was a fellow human being. You just didn't knock them off. No matter how bad it felt. Yes, rights carried responsibilities. And it all depended where you stood what it looked like.

'I think myself - this idea - this idea of a "right to die" is basically a product of our medical and technological advances, ' Roger went on. 'Because we fight so hard to postpone the inevitable end, people now want a right that protects them from our interference. They want to go back, really, back to a state where illness - "natural causes" - could result in a person dying - naturally - in a way they could understand - accept. You know - pneumonia - the old man's friend. That kind of thing.'

'Just the kind of thing my father says. He thinks we've gone too far in some ways - with the technology.'

'I agree - in some ways, I think we have. So it's a rejection of the excessive application of technical skill - postponing death beyond what's reasonable - what's desirable. That's where we've gone too far - at least, in my judgement. You know, we read about these cases - keeping bodies alive by artificially pumping their hearts - whooshing air through their lungs - for years and years. Seems pretty abhorrent to me. I certainly wouldn't want that for myself - or for anyone in my family. No thanks.'

'Nor me.' Ira shuddered.

'So if it's simply that sort of freedom - freedom from excessive intervention - then I think we'd almost all agree. But of course the right to refuse that kind of treatment - that's already enshrined in common law.'

'Uhhm.'

'But it's not quite as simple as that. The modern usage of the term, "right to die" - seems to me, it embraces something more than a right to refuse unwanted treatment. It's a difference of intention really, I suppose. So a second aspect of this so-called "right" involves - involves permitting people to refuse treatment so that they can die. Someone might say, "I will not have any more renal dialysis"; or "I want you to remove this feeding tube". So rather than a choice about how to live while dying - it becomes more a decision about whether to die or to live. Are you with me?'

'Yes. I see that.'

'The next step along the continuum, it seems to me, is a demand for positive assistance - to precipitate the death - speed things up. Here I think perhaps we're talking about a slightly different concept - a "right to be mercifully killed", rather than a "right to die". And here I do have problems.'

'I agree - this bit gives me headaches.'

'But to get back to the business of rights - the sticking point in each situation for me is the corresponding obligation. Do they have a right - a right - to assistance to die? We might choose to give that assistance but I'm not convinced we're morally obliged to give it.'

'Indeed. Actually I'd go further. I'm convinced we're **not**.'

'Well, yes. I think that's my position too. And that's where I feel it's inappropriate to talk about 'rights' in this particular scenario. Because it's not an absolute, unquestionable right. Whatever we might think about the compassionate response to such tragic cases, we can't be held to be

obliged to kill our patients. Not at least if we subscribe to the traditional ethic of medicine - always to care, never to kill. Gosh, Hippocrates would turn in his grave to hear my paraphrase!'

Roger's self mocking tone relieved the tension of Ira's concentration on the thinking behind his words.

Her large dark eyes seemed to look somewhere beyond him even though they were directed at him. Hesitantly she began, 'From the point of view of us - as doctors - I see all that. But I still have this niggling doubt. What about the patient's point of view? What about autonomy and dignity? If a person has a right to exercise control over his own destiny, which I think is a basic right - yes?' Roger nodded. 'Well, couldn't you argue that part of that basic right is choosing the manner and the timing of their death? And with that the right to choose the most humane way to end a life when it's ceased to have meaning or dignity?'

'Good point. If it involves simply stopping treatment - treatment that's become more onerous than beneficial - without prospect of recovery - then I think the person does have the right to choose to stop receiving treatment - to choose not to have a burdensome life unnaturally prolonged. But I still don't quite see that they have the right to oblige someone else to assist them in dying - actively, I mean. You think perhaps they do?'

'Well, no, not exactly. Did you see the interview with the chap with MS last night on TV?' Ira sat forward in her seat, becoming suddenly impassioned. Roger was nodding his head. 'Well, there was this fellow - what was he? - about 50 I'd say. He's had it for 26 years. In a wheel chair - blind. Depends on other people for everything - you know, all the physical care. But, and here's the horror - his mind's bright and alert. He's made a living will that says he wants a way out when he gets to a certain point. Doesn't he have a right to that?'

Roger gave a deep sigh, shaking his head slightly at the thoughts this picture resurrected. 'It's always so much harder when it becomes a personal issue with a real person. I did see that interview, yes, and I felt the strength of his argument. Particularly his point that those folk who say euthanasia should always be illegal should be sitting in his wheelchair. I must admit, I also felt that I'd probably have got to the point of wanting to end it all long before he had. The prospect of being trapped with an alert mind in an unresponsive body, appals me! Infinitely more ghastly than the folk with Alzheimers and so on who don't know what day it is.'

'Me too! But it's odd - it's odd how the breaking point seems to extend - when you actually do get one of these progressive conditions.' Ira sounded almost as if she was speaking to herself. She suddenly looked up from contemplation of her coffee mug. Her voice was curiously flat, unemotional. 'You know that I have MS. Eighteen months now since ...'

'I know. It must have been specially difficult for you - watching that programme.'

'Not as bad as another experience I had recently.' Roger saw the pain in her expression. 'My GP suggested I went to one of these group meeting - you know the sort of thing - 20 or so people all at various stages. Swapping notes and stories. I wished I hadn't gone. It was horrendous - seeing all those people paralysed, dependent, unable to speak clearly. Sort of like seeing yourself in 20 years time - or maybe next year. And not liking what you saw one little bit! I mean, of course you know - you know intellectually what the course of the condition is like, but it's another thing to see it in the raw - and all around you. And to be identifying yourself as one of them. On the same course.'

'You don't need your nose rubbed in it.'

'Exactly. OK some of them said they'd had years and years of normal life in their periods of remission. They'd climbed mountains, skied, had children. Up to now, I've been lucky - but I don't know how quickly my condition will change. And for me - well, I feel it would be quite wrong - totally wrong - to involve other people in risks just because I want to live my life to the full. I mean, just at a fairly basic level - I can just never know when my legs will give out again. It's really frightenening finding you just can't walk or feel your feet.' Ira seemed to have shrunk into herself as she remembered that dreadful fear. Her arms wrapped around her body she rocked slightly, like a troubled child in need of protection from an imagined horror.

'Is that what alerted you, weakness in your legs?' Roger was scanning through what he had just said. Until her reminder he had forgotten she had the disease. He had talked to her simply as a colleague. Had he unwittingly said things which would have made her hurt even worse? So easy to give a quick response and a flip resume - say things you wouldn't say if you were putting yourself in the shoes of the other person - someone with a vested interest. He felt an intense sadness that this lovely young woman should have such a personal investment in a right to die.

'Yes. I was actually getting off a plane home. It was fearfully hot - you know, when we reached Calcutta. I thought - at first - it was simply a reaction to tiredness - excitement - the heat - everything. But I simply couldn't move. Imagine - they had to cart me off on a trolley! Talk about loss of dignity! I didn't even suspect - not that it was anything serious. I actually resisted - quite vocally - resisted being trundled along to the hospital. But my father - he's a neurologist - he insisted. And well, here I am. Diagnosed but mercifully OK - ever since that episode. Shouldn't tempt providence - but ...'

'I'm so sorry - so very sorry.' Roger's sympathy unnerved her more than she had expected. It was so difficult to tell people - well, it wasn't really the telling of the facts, it was facing their kindness, their pity. Strange how it was hardest of all from those people whom you liked best. She admired and respected Roger deeply and the look in his eyes was too much for her composure. She turned away, suddenly intent on the curled end of her thick black plait.

Sensitive to her distress, Roger steered the conversation into generalities to give her breathing space. He wanted to reach out and give this wounded creature a hug but he knew her control was fragile. She would not relish a cathartic reaction at this moment. She was still on duty - had bloods to collect, parents to meet, nurses to relate to. She was not much older than Eleanor. But what a golden future seemed to lie before this Asian girl - beauty, brains, vibrant personality - everything going for her. But blighted by the shadow of this cursed disease. His heart went out to her father. A neurologist! Knowing what he knew about the nerve damage. How could he bear the wanton destruction of this beautiful girl. Cruel, sick world. Eleanor, Ira - what did it all mean?

'Where were we? Ah yes - what we mean by the "right to die". So we seem to be agreed that we sympathise with the patient's right to refuse treatment; his right to choose to stop treatment; his right to be helped to die; his right to control his own dying; his right to a dignified death. But we aren't happy about infringing our own code of morals in order to oblige our patients.'

'Yes, it's a matter of where you're standing.' Ira's voice was low, reflective. She was still hovering between being a patient and being a doctor.

'My feeling is, an already difficult matter is made more complicated when we talk of these things in terms of rights. They sound - too absolute - too immutable. And if I'm honest, I'm uneasy about it. I'm worried that the more radical - the more extreme claims - will be subsumed in the more generally acceptable - because they're presented as extensions of the argument. If you go so far, why not that bit further and then a bit further again? We have to balance the rights of doctors against the rights of patients, I think.'

By now Ira had regained an outward composure. Her intent concentration indicated to the vigilant consultant that she was able to suppress the personal implications sufficiently to be able to grapple with the underlying issues of this thorny problem. It had been a snap decision - this decision to pursue the discussion rather than to abandon the purpose of their meeting because of her painful disclosure. A gamble. Who could ever tell what was right in such situations? There was no right or wrong, merely grey tracks of possibility.

'I see your point.' Ira's voice was steady and strong again. 'Of course there is a special problem for those people who are incurably ill - but with a condition that isn't killing them. You know - slow loss of dignity - loss of function, which is just as unacceptable as the prospect of a lingering death is to, say, someone with cancer. But they can't bring about an end to it as readily - or in ways that won't outrage other people. I mean, if they're physically unable to jump off a high rise block - to get hold of enough drugs - to hold a gun - tie a poly bag round their necks - whatever. Then they're even more disempowered - totally at the mercy of other people's scruples.' Roger could see exactly where she was coming from.

'Absolutely. I have to say, my sense is that it's better left to the compassion and good sense of the medical profession and each individual patient and his family, rather than attempting to enshrine it in law. Once you make a law about it, you set it in concrete. As someone somewhere said, then it's not easily washed out by rain or tears.'

'Exactly. I agree.'

'But, of course, as Britain becomes more and more litigation conscious, you can understand why doctors want some concrete guidelines to back them up. And with the walloping Defence Union subscriptions we all pay, we want some assurance that the courts will give us a reasonable return when things do get nasty. But there speaks an old neonatologist! The fees we pay along with our obstetric friends are not the highest for nothing.' He was warmed by the return of her natural relaxed grin.

'I think the idea of phrasing it in terms of 'rights' is understandable. But I also think this idea has evolved really because of inherent fears,' he went on. 'There are all sorts of fears. There's the fear of life being prolonged - because medical skill and knowledge have advanced to such a degree that it's possible to keep people alive - way beyond the point where simple human kindness says enough is enough. Then there's the fear of living too long - without the old man's friend, pneumonia - or some other fatal disease - to carry us off kindly and naturally. Then there's the fear of senility or loss of dignity. And there's the fear of loss of control - being no longer in a position to determine our destiny, decide what's done with or for our bodies.' Roger ticked each item off on his fingers as he listed the fears.

'And there's another fear,' Ira added. 'The fear of becoming a burden on other people - on your family, on the people you care most about - ruining their lives. And a fear of being a burden on the state. I know I worry about keeping folk alive - you know, the ones that are of no possible present or future value to society - when the money and resources could be better used to certain good for perhaps dozens of others. I know life itself has a value - you can't reduce it to the contribution a person makes to society - but ... It sounds harsh - but it's perhaps less so if I talk about myself again - if you don't mind?' She lifted an eyebrow in enquiry.

'OK. Go ahead.'

'I really don't want vast wadges of money spent keeping me going in a twilight world between living and dying - especially not when I know the same resources could give a vastly better quality of life to several other people - new knees, new hips, perhaps. My mother had a hip replacement - it transformed her life. It's not the dramatic stuff that hits the headlines - but it sure does make life a lot better for folk.'

'Yes. We're very British when it comes to talking about money - too dirty a word to be mixed with medicine. But I take your point. The fear of becoming a burden is another fear I didn't include in my list. But it's very real. We do fear being reduced to a form of person that might make people close to us feel - however they might fight it - feel that they wish we didn't exist. And no matter how much else we might have given them - or can still give them - we could feel our present state is more of a burden than it could ever be of value.'

Ira nodded, dislodging a dark curl from the side of her face which danced with each movement.

'But of course there's the down side of that too - a sort of moral pressure on people not to linger - not to inconvenience or distress those who have to stand by and watch it all.'

'You mean, like from the folk waiting for an aged relative to pop his clogs?'

'Them, yes - and people like hospital administrators - our chief enemies, eh? - worried about cost-cutting yet again!' Ira smiled at his caricature of their economic problems. 'So, I suppose the short answer - after all that - is that I steer away from talking about rights. I do appreciate - fully appreciate - there are times when death is a preferable option to a continuing existence. I suppose I'd go for - prudent discretion - yes, that about describes it - in individual cases.'

'Nice turn of phrase that - prudent discretion.' Ira turned it on her tongue, savouring the concept. 'Yes, I like that.'

'In a nutshell I suppose, leaving aside the issue of rights, my position is this: I defend the practice of allowing patients to die but I oppose the practice of actively and deliberately killing. In Peter's case, I'd be willing to withdraw medical intervention which is stopping him from dying. I would not be prepared to give him a lethal injection to spare us all the agony of the next few hours or days. And you?'

'Much about the same. I feel it's slightly more complicated for me in the case of Peter - compared with a competent adult. I mean I've faced this with an adult patient. OK mostly they can tell you what they want - how they feel. We can't get Peter's views. And the parents - well, it's difficult to know. I think - well, I'm almost certain - most often the parents have got the best interests of the infant at heart. But there's sometimes a nagging feeling that they might - perhaps - sometimes anyway - be overly persuaded by what it means to them rather than what it means to the baby - if he lives or dies.'

'And you feel we should do some more work with the Flanaghan parents - find out just where they stand in this?'

'Yes, I think so. D'you want to do this one yourself? Or d'you want me to talk with them again - bring this up specifically?' Ira tilted her head in enquiry.

'I will, of course, talk with them myself. But any further information you can give - that'd be helpful. If we both get the same messages we're in a stronger position. If they seem to be responding differently to each of us - then I think we'll need to consider - perhaps there's something more complicated going on with this family - more than we yet understand. At the moment I want to know why they're dismissing the idea of discontinuing treatment - without discussion really. The Mum - she seems to think it's God's plan for her. But what about the Dad? Is he simply not ready to contemplate Peter's death? Is he protecting his wife? Has he got a strong religious objection to stopping? Or what is it?'

Roger rose from his seat as he spoke signalling the end to their present discussion.

'Thanks for the chat. You've clearly done a lot of thinking yourself on the main issues. It's helped me - talking to you. We shall try to have another meeting of the team before we do anything - anything irrevocable anyway. But it's certainly helpful to know where each person stands. I've asked Catherine Woollard to sound out her nursing staff and - let's take it from there.'

Ira nodded and prepared to follow him from the room. But he turned back suddenly and with his hand still on the door knob, said quietly, 'If there's anything I can do to help - with your own problems, I mean - please don't hesitate to say. I'm very willing but I don't want to interfere. I'll just take my cue from you.'

'Thank you so much. I appreciate the offer - I'll remember it. But the most helpful thing at the moment is - put it to the back of my mind and everyone carry on as normal.'

'OK. I understand.' Roger's tone and look were gentle and Ira felt a warm reassurance that she could indeed seek this man out if the going got tough.

They had no sooner stepped outside the door than Wendy Greenaway's voice accosted them.

'Oh, there you are, Ira! Labour Ward's just rung. Twins - 23 weeks. Just admitted.'

'Here we go again!' Ira nodded her thanks to Roger and followed Wendy down the corridor. More shuffling of incubators to make room for the coming admissions. Roger watched their retreating forms noting the steady poise of the houseman as she walked. No hint yet of an unstable gait. He devoutly hoped it would be a very long time before there were any outward signs of the coming debility.

A glance at his watch showed him that it was time to keep his appointment with his fellow consultant, Bill Forsyth. He had arranged to discuss Peter's case with Bill and then visit the baby together for a clinical consultation. The third member of the triumvirate, Adrienne Tamworth, was out of the country at the moment but Roger had every intention of consulting her too when she returned. He knew her theoretical position on these matters, but he'd like her view on Peter in particular. He had already reported developments to both of them and shared his concerns about the future of this infant. You had to go over and over the ground - be sure - take account of developments.

Bill was on the phone when Roger arrived at the tiny office he inhabited. Files were piled on every available surface. Transparencies and slides littered the main desk indicating he was in the throes of preparing a lecture. A stained coffee mug and a circle of crumbs on his scribbling block were all that remained of a hasty snack. A large freezer hummed in one corner, its bland exterior giving no clue as to its rather macabre contents. For Bill's consuming interest related to the development of abnormalities in fetuses and the freezer currently contained the bodies of 36 abortuses.

He sat swivelling the chair in which he sat, back and forth, back and forth, idly doodling on the paper around the crumbs, his attention wholly on the conversation. His occasional interjections gave no indication of the content of their discussion so Roger withdrew from the doorway to give him privacy. While he waited, he scanned the notices hung untidily on the board outside Bill's office. Conferences on every conceivable facet of neonatology nowadays. They'd probably all be worth going to but you just couldn't fit in so much time away. The demands of clinical practice and research were so great. Yet another journal starting up - it was hard enough to keep abreast of the ones they had already.

The click of the replaced receiver told him that Bill had concluded the call. His cheery voice bade Roger to enter. 'Hi, there. Sorry to keep you waiting.' Bill's smile was welcoming.

'That's OK. I took the liberty of reading your notices. You going to the Conference in Vienna - the one on respiratory issues? I see the application slip's missing.'

'Thinking of it. Yes. Sent in an abstract last week. If it's accepted, I'll probably go. Makes it more worthwhile - if you give a paper - get a bit of feedback from colleagues.'

Roger nodded, settling himself in the chair opposite Bill's desk.

'What I wanted to see you about today - Peter Flanaghan.'

Bill put his hands together fingertip to fingertip and leaned forward on his elbows.

'Things deteriorated?' he asked.

'Medically speaking, not dramatically. But we aren't winning with this little fellow. He's still on maximum oxygenation and you'll remember he's had a Grade four IVH?'

'Yep. I think I remember the picture. You were concerned about the parents?'

'I was. Still am. Difficult to tell, really. We think they want us to continue. But they aren't really listening to the facts we're presenting. We're thinking of putting the case more strongly - trying to find out what they really want - and why. I'm also consulting everyone else involved. We have some strong feelings amongst the team but, as far as I can tell, it's in control. I'm not expecting problems from that quarter - but of course, you never can tell.'

'Some new blood lately. Haven't got the measure of all of them myself yet. Anyone in particular - giving you headaches, I mean?'

'Bit of strife between the new sister - Wendy? Wendy Greenaway?'

'The Welsh girl? I rather like her. Nice manner. Dedicated sort of girl.'

'Yes. Excellent neonatal nurse. And I agree - friendly, pleasant manner. But strict Catholic - strong views about the sanctity of life.'

'Whoops. Could be trouble.'

'Mmm. Had a bit of a run in with one of the students - at the meeting on Monday.'

'Really?'

'At the other end of the spectrum - this student. Jo Manson. D'you know her? Older girl. You know - bit of a life-not-worth-living-if-you're-handicapped attitude. Has a relative who's pretty severely damaged - from her description. Sounds pretty bitter about it. But certainly no time for "holy" attitudes.'

'So you're monitoring the situation - as they say.'

'That's about it.'

'I'm happy to come down with you - see the notes - have another look at the baby in a bit - if that would help. But what about you? D'you personally feel quite easy about withdrawing treatment - if the parents agree?' Bill's question was quiet but Roger knew he could trust this friend and colleague.

'Well, I never feel comfortable in these cases - but I'm as confident - confident as I could be anyway - that Peter doesn't stand a chance of anything approaching normality. I'd value your opinion, of course. But I'm sure you'll agree with the prognosis.'

'So it's a question of the injury of continued existence?'

'I think so.'

'Well, Rog, I wouldn't presume to tell you what to do on that one. Your own experience gives you the edge every time in my book.' Bill had met Eleanor on several occasions over the years. Roger had consulted him informally over various problems they had had with their only daughter.

'I'm not really into philosophy at all but I was reading something,' Bill was rummaging through an untidy sheaf of papers as he spoke. 'You might be interested. Where is the thing? Saw it this week. Then again you've probably read it. Must be here somewhere.' A cascade of articles slid to the floor further disrupting Bill's filing system. 'One of my students's doing something about - ethics in neonatology. Gave me a copy of this paper. Probably thought I needed bringing up to date.' He paused and then a broad grin spread over his face as he extricated the said paper. 'Ah yes. Eureka!'

He settled himself back in his chair and referred to the document.

'I must say it struck me - hadn't really thought along these lines before. I'm a seat-of-the-pants clinician myself, as you very well know. But anyway - these chaps are basically arguing that abnormal kids don't have any rights. At least - that's my understanding. Seems to me they're saying they aren't persons.'

'Who are the authors?' Roger was leaning forward to see the paper. Bill showed him the article in Archives of Disease in Childhood.

'Know it?'

'I haven't seen that one, no. But odd you should mention it today. I've just been talking with Ira about rights.'

'Ahh - the bold Ira. Bright lassie that one.'

'Indeed.'

'Well, if I can paraphrase - these fellows say having human rights depends on the ability to exercise them. Well, I'm not sure about that. I mean to say - a cactus can bloom in the desert - no one sees it - but it's still there. Just 'cause you can't confirm it doesn't negate its existence - does it?' Bill was hesitant, feeling his way here.

'I see what you mean. There'd be an awful lot of folk who were suspect then. You don't have to be severely abnormal not to be able to exercise your rights, do you?' Roger was in sympathy with his colleague's doubt.

'They sort of deal with that. They say - unless a person possesses a whole list of things - let's see - I've underlined them - self awareness, the capacity to formulate aims and accompanying beliefs, ability to use language, competence to reason, emotional confidence to act and interact with others, and - furthermore - had these capabilities over sustained periods of time - they say it's questionable whether they have human rights. As you say - that includes an awful lot of people!'

'Well, certainly no babies have rights under these criteria. They can't formulate aims, express beliefs, use language, reason, etc. and they have no emotional confidence at all. What's this all about? But I suppose we could say they have potential - potential for personhood - under normal circumstances, I mean. But then there's still a question mark over the Peter Flanaghans of this life.'

'That's exactly how they argue. But these authors - they reckon that if infants are severely mentally and physically disabled, this potential's compromised. But then it seems to me - well, then you run into the problem of deciding at what point - under what circumstances - their human rights can be called into question. I mean - look at our line of work ...'

There was silence. Both men thought ruefully of all those infants they had cared for where there was so much uncertainty - the prognosis was so vague.

'So do we have to treat them as persons - until the evidence proves otherwise? And when we know they'll never be capable of rational thought, then what? How d'you feel about saying, 'Well, they aren't really people after all, so it actually doesn't matter what we do to them' - how about that, Rog?' Bill's mildly scoffing tone showed his disdain for such a thesis. 'Seems fraught with perils to me. But I'm not into that kind of thinking myself - I like to treat them all like persons with rights!' Bill grinned wryly at Roger as he admitted his stance.

'Yes, I exactly see your point. And after all, it all comes down to somebody's evaluation at the end of the day. I've treated Peter Flanaghan as a fellow human being - deserving our best shot, dignity, etc. etc. up until now. So - like you say - at what point do I decide he isn't really a person with rights? No, I accept that's too difficult a notion to apply in practice - no matter how attractive it might be as an argument to moral philosophers.'

Bill was again scanning the paper in front of him.

'That's the trouble with so much of this sort of literature, I find,' Roger sighed. 'Just doesn't seem to hold up in practice.'

'Absolutely. I remember there was one bit - if I can find it - really made me see red. Crazy. Yep, here it is. Listen to this.' Bill was clearly irritated by the arguments of men who didn't seem to understand the world as he saw it. 'They're talking about infants - OK? - our patients now, Rog. The kids we know something about. They list four conditions where they say - these kids - our babies - can never become persons with rights. First one is - let's see - where their condition is terminal and death will pre-empt their potential for future personal development. Second one - is - where they are so mentally retarded through neurological damage that - and I quote - 'the development of self-awareness and intentional action will be virtually impossible'. Third one, dedum, yep, here's number three - they're so severely physically disabled that there's no prospect of them ever being able to act on their own behalf. And the fourth one - if I can find it, deda, deda, deda, ah, yep - where there's very severe physical disability likely - physical disability with accompanying pain and suffering which will entail recurrent invasive treatment. And something about that suffering impairing their autonomy.'

'These chaps are demolishing large sections of our clientele, Bill! Is their contention that we'll find it easier to wipe them out if we adopt their logic?'

'Not quite! But I do still have a problem with this whole notion - you know - saying they aren't persons. I mean - it just wouldn't work - not in clinical practice. Would it?'

'No - I don't see how we could apply those sorts of criteria. It'd be horrific - and mightily confusing to boot.'

'And that's exactly what the neonatologist commenting on this paper concludes. It was a great relief to read what he had to say, I must admit. He reckons the idea of them not ever being persons with rights would stick in the throats of most paediatricians who regularly see severely handicapped children.'

'So you and I are not so amateurish after all!' Roger laughed. 'I don't know - it can be irritating. But maybe it's useful - exploring the basic principles. But in practice - you and I - we see such a vast range of individuals. Everything's not buttoned up and watertight - not in real life. I'm frankly doubtful. Don't see that trying to draw up set guidelines could ever be sufficiently - I don't know - robust? - flexible? - comprehensive enough? - to take account of all the permutations of real life. All the different families - how they respond. Could I read that paper at some point, please?'

'Of course. I'll photocopy it for you.' Bill stuck a yellow Post-it on the paper and scribbled an indecipherable message to himself.

The two men then walked downstairs to the Unit. They spent some time with Peter, examining his fragile body, percussing, feeling, listening, watching, thinking. Grave faced, they withdrew to the office to consult his records. Bill had no qualms about confirming Roger's prognosis. Perched on the edge of the desk, the door closed, they talked about the options - the timing - the sequence of events - recording consultations - involving the parents.

Roger felt reassured by Bill's confirmation of his intentions and the two men parted in mutual sympathy. So many times they had individually faced this grim task. It did not get easier. It always grieved Roger that people could imply that neonatologists were so casual about these matters - regarded their patient's lives as of little value - dispensible. It was never like that. He sighed deeply. There were some heavy sessions ahead. It all took its toll.

CHAPTER 8

The Flanaghans' Dilemma

For Sue and Richard Flanaghan the days dragged slowly by in a daze of dulled pain and suspended animation. They went through the motions of sustaining their ordinary lives, but the events in the Neonatal Unit eclipsed any other consideration. Teaching, cooking, conversing, housework - everything seemed so unimportant somehow. It was hard even to give Victoria the attention she normally received and both parents were glad that she was now happily ensconsed with her favourite grandparents. She'd probably come back utterly ruined but perhaps that was a reasonable trade-off. At least for the time being she was the centre of someone's attention.

Peter's precipitate and early birth had shocked them deeply. Both were committed Christians, regular church-goers. They had clung to their beliefs - in the bad times as well as the good. Life was divinely ordained. But sometimes it was hard to see where God was taking them.

Endlessly they had relived events leading up to that first ominous contraction, searching for some acceptable explanation. Finding nothing to satisfy their intellects they reviewed their wider lives. Were they being singled out for special punishment? Whom the Lord loveth he chasteneth. The gnawing sense of guilt haunted Sue's waking hours - the conviction grew that she was in some way to blame for this calamity. She must accept the retribution. God was teaching her something - she didn't know what. Perhaps it was because she put her family first - ahead of God. Perhaps it was that she took such a pride in her home, loved material things too much. Perhaps her occasional feelings of envy or coveting other people's new car or foreign holiday were enough to show God she needed a refining experience. There was plenty she could find to criticise in her life. She schooled herself to accept the correction irrespective of the sin. God knew best.

Richard listened patiently to her wonderings. Again and again he reassured her that she wasn't wicked or evil. Over and over again he told her what a perfect wife and mother she had always been. How much he loved her. Vaguely she noticed that he didn't ever seem to blame himself. So it must be her fault. The soul searching had to continue.

It was now five and a half weeks into the experience. The three hours they had spent in the nursery had unnerved Sue. Peter seemed so ill, so unresponsive. And she had hated the suggestion that it might not be in his own interests to be kept alive. It wasn't for mere mortals to decide such things. If it was in the divine scheme of things that he should live - then who were they to think they knew better? If he was meant to die he would die in spite of all the technology, all the skill.

Normally she worked hard at being composed - for Richard's sake. He was always so supportive. She didn't want to make things harder for him. He hated her being upset. Today she could maintain the pretence no longer.

'I thought God had punished me enough when Briony died,' she sobbed. 'Life seemed so awful - I wanted to die myself. I even - I even went to the river - I just wanted to end all the misery - stop all the hurting. I thought - maybe it was - 'cos I was so - unworthy. Maybe - if I wasn't there - it would all work out. But I couldn't do it - not when it came to it - I just couldn't. I just knew - I've always known - it's a mortal sin - taking your life - I couldn't do it.'

Richard moved swiftly to take her in his arms rocking the crumpled body, soothing, dropping kisses on the fair hair.

'Thank God you didn't! I couldn't have borne to lose you too,' his muffled voice was hoarse at the prospect.

'Oh, Richard, I miss her so much. I only feel complete when I go to talk to her.'

'When you what?' Richard froze.

'When I go to talk to her - to Briony - to her grave. I sit there - talk to her.'

'I didn't know you did that.'

A cold hand gripped Richard's heart. He felt excluded, shut out by the one person who meant more to him than life itself.

'I couldn't tell you. I thought - you expected me to be over it - and - and you hardly ever - mention her now.' Sue's explanation was broken by her shuddering sobs. But a torrent of pent-up emotion had been released. 'I thought you'd forgotten - or at least - it didn't hurt now - to remember. So I thought - you wouldn't like it - if you knew - I was still feeling - so bad. Oh Richard - I do feel so - miserable. It hurts - so much. I - miss her - all the time. I don't feel - any better - than when it - it first happened. The books - all say time - heals, - the counsellors - tell you - the pain turns into - gentler memories, but - it's not true - it's not - it's not - not for me. It hurts - so much still - like a physical pain. I think - God is - punishing me - for loving Briony so much - maybe more than - I love Him.'

Richard was aghast at the tortured expression in his wife's eyes. He had had no idea she felt like this.

'You should have told me!' he protested.

'And you wouldn't - have told me to - pull myself together - be brave - look forward - not back?'

He had the grace to look ashamed.

'Well, OK, I might have said something like that.'

'But I can't, Richard, I can't pull myself together about this. It's just - too painful - too deep a pain. It will take - it's not a matter - of - willpower. I can't really explain it but it's like - like as if a bit of me died with Briony. And I only get that bit back when I'm close to her - feel her nearness, talk to her. I know it sounds as if I'm going off my trolley but I'm not - I don't think anyway!' Her weeping was abating as she brought all her fears out for him to share.

'You're not. You're not,' he reassured her tightening his arms about her.

'And that's why - partly anyway - why I can't bear to think we might lose Peter. I can't cope with another bit of me dying. Oh, I know it's different. We haven't got to know him as a real little person like Briony. He hasn't been sitting in this chair, reading a favourite book, reaching up chubby little arms to hug you and say, "I love you, Mummy". Not like Briony. But it's harder in other ways. I mean - biologically he's a bit of me. I carried him inside me all those weeks; sheltered him, cherished him. Felt his kicking, his stretching. Watched him being born - emerging from my own body. How can I bury him in the ground - walk away to a life without him? Richard, I can't do it! I can't.' Tears streamed down her blotched face as she buried her head in his shoulder.

'I know. I know.' Rocking her fiercely he tried to blot out the memories of that other funeral suddenly so vivid, of the moment when they'd found Briony.

It had been a normal Saturday excursion to visit his brother's home. Briony was playing with her four older cousins - the adults lazily gossiping, drinking in the sun and fruit punch on the patio. The carefree laughter from the terraced garden mingled with the drone of Carl's bees - peaceful, secure. Scampering feet rushed to hide - loud countdowns -tentative calls as the seeker sought those hidden forms. Suppressed giggles gave the game away for the youngest ones. Exaggerated shrieks from the older ones as they were discovered kept the excitement high. It was hot work. The three eldest cousins clamoured for liquid refreshment. Sue and her sister-in-law, Kate, brought long cold drinks. They drank thirstily. Flopped on the grass - temporarily grounded.

Richard had been half asleep on the sun lounger, a newspaper protecting him from youthful interference. It was only when the children suggested a game of rounders that Sue asked whether it wasn't time to 'find' the two younger children. Puzzled protests followed. They'd finished the game of hide and seek ages ago. Briony and Graham? Gone in search of bits and pieces to make a garden on a plate. Weren't they indoors making the creations? No. Then they must still be in the bottom part of the garden searching for treasures.

It was Sue who found Briony face down in the pond. Her screams roused the neighbourhood to activity. But Briony was beyond their vigorous and frenzied attempts at resuscitation. Stunned silent horror gave way to lashing recriminations. Who had been looking after her? Why did they leave her? Why wasn't the pond better protected? Why had they come?

Sue wouldn't put the wet body down. Clutched it close, speechless, wild eyed, unbelieving. Richard so much wanted to comfort her. She pushed him away. No-one - nothing could help.

Richard had carried the little white coffin himself. He had had to steel himself to think of mechanical movements, where to stand, where to look, to hold himself together. He couldn't think of what they were really doing as the cruelly small box was lowered into that yawning hole. Instead he worried - fretted about Sue. His brother told him - afterwards. He was like a hen fussing, hovering. But he couldn't help himself - he was overwhelmed by the strength of his own feelings. He couldn't bear that Sue - his beloved Sue - should hurt like that. Hurt so much, there was no room for him.

Life went on - everyone said so. And they commended his strength, bearing it so bravely. They weren't to know he had papered over the raw hurt with a veneer shutting out emotion, not acknowledging his grief, his fear, lest it overwhelm him. He knew, and his GP suspected, that the spate of ailments he's suffered subsequently had been due to his suppressed emotions. Other people sympathised with his 'run of bad luck' and admired his fortitude.

When her sobbing had abated somewhat, Sue ventured a question.

'Richard, how would you - really feel - about Peter being terribly handicapped?'

He was a long time replying and when it came his answer was slow and somehow flat, devoid of feeling.

'I don't know. I suppose my biggest anxiety is for you. You get worn out with just looking after Victoria. I hate to see you so tired - exhausted. And she's perfectly normal - does so much for herself. How would you cope with Peter - a child who always needs everything doing for him? Demands attention all day, all night? Never really grows up. He'd get more difficult to care for as you get older - less able to lift and bend.'

'You speak as if I'd be on my own. Wouldn't you help?'

'Well, of course I would - if I could. But I have to go out to work - you know how much I'm involved in everything - extra curricular activities, meetings, societies, everything - got to be. Can't afford to slack - got to hold on to the job. We can't manage without an income, can we? I'd help - of course I would - when I could. But the bulk of the work - that'd fall on you.'

'I can do it, I know I can! I'll be given the strength.' She was suddenly animated. 'And Victoria will help me.'

'Is that fair on her?'

'Fair? No, of course it isn't! None of this is fair! Nobody ever said life was fair!'

He was startled by her vehemence. She moved now to free herself from his arms. Turning in her seat she looked directly into his dark eyes and in a low hard voice asked, 'Are you suggesting - we should let them turn off the machine?'

'I'm not suggesting anything. Not yet. It's too soon. I'm simply trying to think it all through. You must have heard Dr Carshalton - probing, sounding us out. They - the doctors - they're considering - whether or not to continue.'

'Of course I heard! But it's different for them. They do this kind of thing all the time. They aren't their babies. Peter is our baby. Our only son. You and I, we made him. He's a part of us. We couldn't - couldn't - turn our back on him!

'I know. I know. What about him though? D'you want him to have pain, suffering all his life? What about the indignity he'll have to endure being cared for - all his days? And even so - he might - he might die - in a couple of years time. Will it be any easier - losing him when he's grown up?'

'I'm surprised at you! Where's your faith? God won't allow him to be tested beyond what he can bear - the Bible says so. And anyway maybe - well, maybe he won't be so badly disabled - not as bad as they think. They're often wrong. You hear all the time - people do much better than they think - get better, live longer, do more than they thought they ever would. You'll see! Peter'll grow up to be a son you can be proud of yet. We can do it - together - with God's help. We can. And Mum and Dad, they'll help us. They will.' The confident ring in her voice and her 'missionary zeal' disturbed him deeply but he could not bring himself to let her see his own great doubts, his wavering faith. Instead he enveloped her once again in a strong embrace murmuring, 'You're incredible, you know that?'

How devoutly he wished he could echo her sentiments. Until the tragedy with Briony he'd believed too. The same simple naive faith. Believed it all worked together for good for those who loved God. He'd learned the verses off pat too. But it didn't add up. Not any more. All the suffering - all the injustice. How was it working for good? OK you heard of these families where they had a death, a handicapped child, somebody who took drugs, went to prison - and it brought new meaning into their lives. Sue had lots of books - the ones the parents wrote. Saying how they'd seen the light. He'd dipped into them - when Sue had coaxed him - but he hadn't been moved. Too sentimental. Not for him. Just their way of coping he reckoned.

OK there probably was a God - he'd go that far. Perhaps he needed to believe there was something, someone out there - in control. But it seemed unlikely that He intervened - interfered - in the little things that happened. What did he think this God did? Difficult one. Probably it was all to do with what believing did for you. It gave you the strength to cope with all the difficult times. He'd had his problems. Had God put them there? Probably not. Had He taken them away? No. Peter was still fighting for his life. Briony was still dead. Sue was still shutting him out of a part of her life and love. His mother was still making him shudder and pretend.

He couldn't even echo Sue's conviction that the grandparents would help. OK, her parents - they would. Brilliant they were. But not his. He couldn't even suggest it. She wouldn't know that - that was his secret.

Holding her, savouring the fragrance of her hair, the softness of her body in his arms, he remembered his own discovery. He had never been close to his father. A weak and ineffectual man, Father, dominated by his wife. Publicly, continually denigrated - humiliated at every opportunity. So used to it he wore a permanent air of apology. Richard remembered lying in bed at night - hearing the sound of their mother's rages - splitting the evening peace. Hunching up the bedclothes - trying - trying desperately to block it out. Struggling to sleep - courting oblivion. Curt creeping into his bed when the crashing started. Holding each other tight. Silent. Unable to speak this horror even brother to brother.

Growing older they learned to drown the nightmare noises with radio and tape. Not even a shared bed now to ease the fear. A conspiracy of silence. It was as if it never was. The revelation had come to them both simultaneously. At breakfast one Thursday morning it had dawned. Father had a great bruise under his right eye. He sat down very gingerly. Winced when he drank his orange juice. The two boys had sat stunned - staring. Unable to believe what their minds told them. Mother - their mother - a battering wife? Couldn't be. It happened in other homes - the lower classes. Not to the Flanaghans. Decent, upright citizens. Middle class. Good neighbourhood. But they knew. Deep down they knew.

They came to be glad that her aim was good. It was rare that the damage was visible. They could conceal the truth as long as their father could conceal the evidence. He never ever betrayed by so much as a flicker what had transpired but his efforts at concealment seemed to seal his emotions and stultify his powers of communication. He was unavailable to his children.

Richard fought against his feelings. It was beyond his comprehension why his father stayed - why he colluded in the concealment. But in spite of himself he loved his mother. Oh he hated what she did. But she was good to him. Rarely ever lost her temper with him or with Curt. It was almost as if she got rid of all her frustration, irritation, anger on her husband, freeing her to be calm and reasonable with her children. But everything was coloured by their apprehension - their fear - that she would betray them in public. Richard remembered the sick feeling - the sneering, the derision, the scorn - her looks, her actions. Remembered wondering what other people made of this couple. Wondering what they would think - if they knew - what he and Curt knew. He shuddered now at the memory.

The movement made Sue turn her head to look up at him.

'Someone walking over my grave,' he quipped. He forced himself to smile and bent to kiss her. Her response eased the hurt of the earlier exclusion. With a sigh she nestled back against his shoulder. He tightened his hold, his face close against hers.

The peace of this shared moment gave him the courage to return to his youth. The security of the love of this woman enabled him to deal with his past fears. He had moved out as soon as he could after finishing school. How he had revelled in the independence of college life. No-one to disturb his peace. Trips home had become less and less frequent - he began to take in the enormity of what the earlier years had done to him. But they had given him a distrust - a distrust of women. He had felt the inadequacy - seen it reflected in the eyes of his first few girlfriends. He knew they'd been mystified - perplexed by his cautious timidity. Somehow he hadn't been able to establish himself as a romantic partner - more of a convenient escort to college events and the local hostelry. They soon got tired of him - left him more distrusting - more unsure.

Sue had been in the same year at University, shared some of the same tutorials and lectures. It had been their common interest in religion that threw them together initially. How he had enjoyed their stimulating debates long into the evening - all those heady nights in third year. She had caught him unawares. Disguised by all this intellectual clothing, their developing relationship had crept up on him subtly, unobserved. He realized with a shock - he couldn't stop thinking about her. He was deeply in love with her before he realized his emotions had been touched. There had been no time to erect his defences. No tentative dates - no expectations. Just a natural easy friendship - but one that had now got out of hand.

He had frozen - appalled. Avoided her. Kept to his room. After ten days - ten miserable lonely days, she had appeared one evening - appeared at his door. Her big eyes - bewildered - questioning - they'd unnerved him. She'd been perfectly direct. Why was he avoiding her? What had she done?

What could he say? Tell her he was scared - of her? Of women? No, there was no explanation. He'd mumbled something. She had overridden his excuses. She'd missed his company. His heart missed a beat. Was it possible ...? No, she couldn't feel the same - wouldn't be here now being so direct - so uncomplicated. She was keen to pick up where they'd left off - discussing the merits of Kant's theories. He was instantly involved in her latest literary find.

Ashamed of his reaction in the face of her candour and forgiving friendship, Richard had re-entered the relationship. But now he was vigilant - kept a closer guard on his emotions. He'd actually welcomed the four week break over Christmas. He'd gone home for the whole of the period. Mother's violence seemed somehow safer - safer than this continued onslaught on his heart.

Then there'd been the invitations - to Dumfries - to meet her family. Far too significant. He wasn't ready for that sort of thing. But in the end he'd run out of plausible excuses. Their genuine unquestioning welcome charmed him. No overtones. No innuendoes. He'd drunk greedily of the calm of this ordinary home. He remembered the thrill of lying awake at night, relaxed, savouring the quiet. No raised harsh voice, no thuds. Simply the friendly quiet of a peaceful home.

The contrast with his own domestic heritage - that had bothered him next. Sue seemed so pure - so thoroughly untouched by anything remotely unsavoury. He'd watched her in church - out of the corner of his eye - lost in the solemnity, the peace of morning worship. Looked untouchable - almost holy. He'd recoiled from the thought of her ever being exposed to the full horrors of home life at it existed for him. He'd had to concoct elaborate reasons for not returning her invitation. Deceit. Half truths. All to protect her.

Safe in the anonymity of college life, he could relax again. Marvel at the blossoming of her love for him. He became fiercely protective, totally absorbed in this lovely creature. She made him feel at once a god and a man; ecstatically happy and profoundly fearful. It had been a spur of the moment thing with him - the proposal. They were sitting beside the lake. The moon fragmented in the ripples they made with skimming stones. He knew with sudden certainty that he wanted this girl - more than he had wanted anything ever before - wanted to spend the rest of his life with her. He had almost blurted it out - stuttered, unrehearsed. Sue had behaved as if he had delivered a Shakespearean soliloquy. Her simplicity - the essential uncomplicatedness - stirred him anew. He shuddered inside at the prospect of her knowing his dark secret.

It was perhaps this crystallising of his fear - he would never allow himself to analyse his motives - that prompted him to propose that they simply cut all the flummery and nonsense - go off and got married - then tell the families. He'd been single-minded about it. Hadn't stopped to ask questions. Had Sue dreamed of a fleet of bridal cars, floating lace veil, and a three-tiered cake? Would her parents be disappointed? Could they afford it? Only one thing mattered. They wanted to be together, didn't they? Why wait? Now they'd made their commitment, they might as well seal it straight away. It was only afterwards - when he'd allowed himself to look again at that time - that he knew he had had an ulterior motive too. Rapt in her own glow of happiness Sue had conceded. That was one of the lovely things about her - the way she looked to him for guidance. She made him feel powerful, protective, strong. Strong enough for both of them. Within two weeks she had acquired a new ivory dress and had become Mrs Richard Flanaghan.

If she wondered at not being introduced to her parents-in-law, she never said so. At first she'd been so busy - busy turning their tiny rented flat into a home. Cooking, cleaning, sewing, mending - all with the same enthusiastic vigour she brought to her studying. With major exams looming neither of them had space for worrying overly about priorities in the entertaining stakes. But it had preyed on Richard's mind - the oddness of their not meeting. Didn't want her getting suspicious. It was exactly four months after their wedding that he had nonchalantly suggested they invite his parents to tea - let them meet their new daughter. He'd felt like a hypocrite - Sue had been so delighted at the prospect - set to work to conjure up a gourmet meal out of student pickings.

The feeling of relief had been even more powerful than the anticipatory fear. The event had passed off with no major embarrassment. His own tension had robbed him of his appetite - stultified his conversation. Sue had teased him - afterwards - teased him for being so uncertain a master in his own house. She was proud to be his wife - he should be confident, assured - a thoroughly married man - keeping his own household. Hadn't he been proud of their entertaining skills? If only she knew!

He stirred now to change his hold of her. He had always been proud of her - always. He'd been rather in awe of her - her steady calm, her unwavering faith. That made her present distress the more disturbing. What had changed?

When he'd acquired an excellent degree - gone into teaching - she'd been an enthusiastic supporter. She had revelled in his success, his popularity. Confirming him as deserving of all the accolades he received. Glad for him - with him. When she had been unable to get employment at first - she'd been calm, patient. He remembered. He'd been so impressed. She didn't sit around moping, downcast. Applied herself energetically to converting their new semi-detached into an attractive and welcoming home. The job with a publishing firm had been just a job - not really what she wanted. But she'd been philosophical. The money would help. And it was only till the children came along. Yes, he'd always been proud of her. She had always had this quiet conviction - everything worked together for good ... She lived it. In the peace - the happiness of those early years he had been persuaded too. God was in His heaven - all was - it definitely was - right with the world. Even keeping his mother at a distance got easier. They settled into a comfortable - well, familiar anyway - a familiar habit of one brief visit every three months - always on Richard and Sue's territory.

The years had rolled by. But the longed-for children didn't follow. Sue had impressed him again. Calmly accepted 'God's will' - explored the possibility of adoption. They had been so fortunate - was it fortune? luck? God's plan for them? Who knew? Babies were scarce commodities. But Briony was available - what an inappropriate term to use! That's what they'd said - there's a little girl available ... He recalled Sue's breathless phonecall - the trip to the house to see her with her foster parents. Worrying about their feelings letting her go - go for good - to a new home - their home. Oh, they needn't worry - she'd be treasured - like their very own. Briony had come into their lives at the age of 18 months. She nestled straight into their hearts with her endearing ways. Sue was transformed. No longer a slightly ill at ease cog in the publishing machinery - now a confident mother reigning supreme in her daughter's affections. The two became inseparable.

Relaxed, happy - she'd been delighted when, three years after Briony's arrival, she'd found herself pregnant. Their cup had run over with joy.

They had laughed and cried and drunk champagne for breakfast - to celebrate. Only a drop for Sue - she wasn't taking any chances. Not with this precious baby. He had guarded her tenderly - taking on some of her tasks - cossetting her, protecting her. For another three months they had gloried in the perfection that life handed them. Then - in an instant - with one cruel blow - their world had been shattered. Briony's accident defied them to find the good - challenged their faith - rocked their confidence. Sue endlessly blamed herself for not having taken better care of this treasure God had given her. Richard withdrew - shocked by the complexity of his emotions. He grieved too - deeply - silently. But Sue was always his number one girl. It was for her pain he grieved, more even than for his own loss. And - he pushed away the thought - but a little bit of him acknowledged it - he was glad in one way. Glad to have Sue all to himself again. Her undivided love. Like it used to be. Except that it wasn't. It wasn't like it used to be. There was the shadow of Briony between them. And until today that shadow had been vague - unspoken.

Back then, it had been a joint effort. Trying to put the fragments together - deal with the pain - prepare for the new baby. The excitement had gone out of the preparation. Richard had been there - at the birth. He saw the look on Sue's face when they said it's a girl. Bitter-sweet. Another girl. He'd felt so powerless seeing her weeping - often. He could only dimly understand it. But he knew he'd got it wrong - the day he took one of

Briony's dresses and put it on Victoria. Sue had been beside herself. She'd railed against his insensitivity. How could he have done it? To imagine for one instance that Briony was back. He was bewildered. Imagined? He hadn't imagined anything. It had been a simple mistake. He'd taken the offending garment from the wrong drawer. But something in him shrank from this new Sue - this person who had raw nerves which he could touch unwittingly. He could now cause her a pain he was powerless to guard against. This girl whom he loved so passionately - he was suddenly a danger to her.

Although she loved Victoria fiercely, Sue had lost the bloom she had had with Briony's growing up. She was nervous - much more fractious than before. Her fanatical attention to Victoria's manners and appearance worried him - seemed to symbolise eternal efforts to assuage an unspeakable guilt, to compensate for an unimaginable failure. Reminded him of psychology lectures - the ones about people who repeatedly washed their hands. Washing away guilt.

Richard had immersed himself more and more in school activities throughout the early days - those terrible weeks after Briony's death. It was only there that he could blot out the pain for any length of time. The very sight of Sue's tragic face undid him. He tried - oh how hard he tried - to take an interest in the pregnancy. But there was this great fear - enveloping him - crushing his sincerity - even as he mouthed the words. If something so appalling could happen once, why not a further disaster? He dared not let himself hope - what would he hope for? - an uneventful delivery - a perfect child. By the time Sue eventually went into labour - after three false starts - he had steeled himself. Convinced himself that there was something far wrong with this new baby. Even checking her physical perfection for himself - counting the perfect fingers and toes - he was sceptical. Doubting, like Thomas - not daring to believe. What about her mental acuity? It'd be a long time before they knew if she was mentally impaired. No point in hoping prematurely.

Deliberately, he had held himself back from forming too close an affection for his daughter. That way he wouldn't be so hurt when things went wrong. But his careful logic had not bargained on the wheedling ways of the very young. Once again he lost his heart to charm and trust.

As the bright and inquisitive toddler reached the milestones expected of her age and maturity - only then had he dared to hope. Gradually, consciously, he let the fears recede. But they were both - he and Sue - both constantly vigilant this time around. People wanted to babysit - no, thanks all the same. They needed to know first hand - Victoria - their precious daughter - only daughter now - was safe, alive. Were people's feelings tramelled? Too bad. Something much more important at stake here. They rarely went out anywhere. The enforced confinement threw them together even more. They depended on each other utterly.

He felt again the sinking feeling he'd felt all those years ago when the phone call came. It had been his mother. They were moving. Nearer to Richard and Sue - and the baby. No explanation, just the information. They'd bought the house and would be moving in three months time. He had wanted to scream at her to stay away and leave him in peace. But he didn't. It had kept him awake at night - worrying, scheming. He had to keep them away - keep Sue from a knowledge of the truth. The family skeleton had to remain buried. How cruel, how hurtful - some of these trite sayings.

Richard's attention was dragged into the present by Sue stirring. She'd get them both a cup of tea. Companionable. Ordinary. Everyday. It helped. He watched her leave the room - slim, graceful. Marvelled at the feelings she kept alive in him - in spite of all the troubles. He couldn't break her heart by telling her the truth - the truth about his beliefs.

He groaned as he leaned back on the settee, closing his eyes, reliving the end of his hope. It had been the period of subdued fears that had brought Peter into being. Funny that - the difference anxiety made to conceiving. And he'd relaxed too - maybe God did care - maybe He'd sent Victoria to soothe their wounds. She had - she certainly had made things better.

Then it was all wiped out. All the benefit of the doubt - all destroyed. Capricious. Unfair. Unjust. No thanks - a God like that - not for me. He had to go and wreck everything. But why? Why them? Did He take some kind of malicious delight - watching them squirming in agony, powerless, puny? Did He get a kick out of seeing that ghastly unfinished form struggling for every breath in the nursery? Was He testing their faith, presenting them with this horrendous dilemma - threatening their marriage, their future, their confidence in Him? Would He punish them if they got it wrong - decided on a course of action He didn't think was for their own good? Richard's fevered imagination tormented him.

His rebellion was the harder to bear because it had to be suppressed. Sue's faith remained unwavering. He was awed by her unquestioning acceptance - her humility. And that of her parents. They remained as devout as always. Supporting her. Confirming her conviction. And that's what she wanted. What he couldn't give her. It grieved him that she turned elsewhere for anything. She was everything for him - he wanted nothing, no-one else. And he needed it to be the same for her. But for now - until they returned to that state - now he couldn't add to her burdens. He couldn't worry her with his spiritual well-being - or lack of it - on top of everything else. It would be too cruel. But he could rebel - secretly - rail against Peter's Creator. He could - and he did.

He opened his eyes, focusing on the room again - scene of so many family moments. There on the mantelpiece was the blurred polaroid photo. The only one of Peter. All they had here to prove he existed. The clarity lost through the perspex of the incubator. But there - in pride of place. Pride? - he felt no pride. Just an emptiness. How could their love have produced such a travesty of a human being?

Where would it all end? What was the right decision? His first thought was always Sue. What was right for her - best for her? He couldn't bear the thought of her wearing out with the struggle. Better a clean break now - better than years of sorrow and pain. Better than the agony of losing Peter later - when she'd grown closer, more fond of him. And Victoria? They had something strong and good with Victoria. Would it survive? Survive sharing her mother with a totally dependent brother? Survive her mother's exhaustion? Survive the necessity for her to take her share, caring for him - as he grew up, became more of a liability, more of an embarassment? And what about her friends - boyfriends? Who'd want to know? Who'd want to run the risk of marrying into a family where they had horribly deformed kids? And who'd want to take on the burden of a severely disabled man when he and Sue had gone? Not even his sister probably. Who could blame her. His mind raced ahead. He shuddered as his imagination pictured the struggles.

Then what about his own interests? Richard forced himself to face the truth. Deep inside he knew. He knew he'd been fighting an unarticulated battle within himself - for years. He acknowledged it now - now in this moment of deep soul searching - seeking for an answer. The truth? The truth was he resented the children - he resented the huge love Sue felt for them. The special bond that excluded him. Even in the midst of his joy in having two little girls to father - he had felt the stirrings. The jealousy. Seen them as rivals for her time and love. In the depths of his grief for Briony, he had yet revelled in Sue's undivided attention once again. The infertile years, the months when they had stayed close at home guarding Victoria's vulnerable years - they had brought them very close. No intrusions - no-one to divert the attention of either elsewhere.

He loved her with a passion and an intensity that scared him. That she returned his love - he had never got over the wonder of that. Because of his mother, his fear of women - it had been the more precious. The way she loved him - unreservedly. He had been the centre of her universe - once. Before the children. Sue had more than made up for all the early damage. But he wanted her, needed her, totally.

She returned to the room now, with a tray of tea and shortbread and her lovely smile. Dropping down on her knees on the floor beside him, she rested her head against his knee, holding her mug in both hands as if she were cold. He leaned back, watching the flickering light casting moving shadows on her features.

'Lovely. I was ready for a cuppa.'

'Me too.'

No, he couldn't break this fragile heart by telling her he wanted them to switch off the ventilator. Instead he suggested, 'Why don't we have another talk with the doctors tomorrow? Let them guide us.'

'They're still going to ask us what we want. I know what I want - I want Peter. But I don't know what you want. You haven't said.'

Richard was glad she kept her eyes on the fire.

'I've been sitting here thinking about it - what's best for him - best for you - best for Victoria. I need more facts.' The excuse sounded lame even to him as he caressed her soft hair.

'You know, Wendy - the short sister with the curly hair - Welsh accent?'

'Yes.' He knew Wendy. Liked her. Felt most comfortable with her.

'Well, she's a staunch Catholic - doesn't believe any life should be cut short. All life is sacred. Even imperfect ones like Peter's. I like that idea. Even those tiny babies who aren't going to live very long, she says, they have a right to be here too - they're precious - no-one has the right to shorten their lives except God.'

Sue had been so comforted by Wendy. With all her experience, she believed. It felt good - entrusting their baby to someone who cared like that. Thought he was so special. Some of them - OK they were technically competent - Peter was safe. But they didn't care - well, not like Wendy cared. And you could talk to her - about God, about faith, about the purpose of it all. You didn't feel embarrassed, awkward. Because she understood. It was important to her too.

Inwardly Richard cursed Wendy for her views.

'But I get the impression the doctors don't think that,' he countered.

'But do you? That's more to the point. What do you think?'

'Well, no, I suppose I wouldn't go quite that far.' Richard spoke slowly, weighing his words. Steering a path between truth and diplomacy. Wanting to protect her. 'The way I see it - when somebody has cancer, say, and they're in agony, I don't think it's humane to let them go on and on suffering. I think you should give them enough painkillers - enough to stop the suffering. If that shortens their life, well, so what? Better two weeks of decent life than four weeks of absolute misery. Well, I think so anyway.'

'But sometimes people are - refined by suffering - become finer people. It brings out their best qualities - what about that? Wendy thinks so. She's seen it happen. And I've read about it - you know. My books.'

Sue remembered Wendy's words. 'It takes time. Sometimes people don't want to face it. They rebel. But time helps. They get a better perspective. They see a different side of it. God helps them see the real values - not the ones they've always thought were important. But the unseen things. The things that make for real peace - lasting happiness. Bigger than the little experiences we have - in this life.'

Now she added her own thought. 'Maybe if you don't give them time - if you shorten the suffering - they won't get to that point that God wanted them to.'

'You're too nice a person by half for this ugly old world,' Richard diverted the question lest he betray his real conviction. 'There aren't nearly as many people who will be 'refined' as you put it, as there are people who will swear and rebel and turn against God. I haven't heard of too many deathbed conversions in real life. And those I have been told about, make me wonder. D'you not think they're just hedging their bets? You know, nothing-to-lose, everything-to-gain - that kind of idea?'

'What an old sceptic!' her tone was teasing.

'Maybe. Perhaps I'm just getting older and wiser! Less gullible!'

A brief smile lit up her face momentarily. As the shadows reappeared, she asked, 'To get back to Peter then, you want us to talk to the doctors again - see if they can help us weigh up the options?'

'That's what I'd do. But what d'you feel about that? D'you think it's a waste of time - because you've already made up your mind?'

'No. It's not a waste of time. Not if that will help you to see he has a chance.'

He knew she had made up her own mind on this - irrevocably. His suspicion had solidified into certainty two days ago. They had been to her parents for a meal and to spend time with Victoria. When it came to the child's bedtime, she had clung to her mother weeping.

'Don't go, Mummy. Mummy, I don't want you to go.'

Granny Flanaghan would not do. Much loved, devoted as she was, she was not Mummy. The child's cries became shriller.

Sue took her upstairs, rocking, crooning, soothing. She sat in the huge cushioned windowseat in her own old bedroom, cradling the distraught child, fighting above the shrieks to calm her fears. At first the strenuous struggles took all her strength. But gradually, almost imperceptibly, the reassurances had their effect. The noise abated, the eyelids drooped, the damp head slumped against the mother's breast. Sue continued to rock, soothing her own frayed nerves as well as those of the drowsy child.

Much later Richard had crept up to see how Sue was faring. As he trod softly across the landing he heard Sue's voice. He stopped - eavesdropping.

'So, you see, my darling, it's not that I don't love you. I do. More than I can ever tell you. I love you and Peter more than anyone else in the whole world. You're both my special people - my babies.' Richard froze. What had begun as an innocent and loving intrusion into Sue's privacy, now took on dark overtones.

'But God has chosen us to have a very special baby to look after. He's chosen you too, to help look after him. I know we can do it if we all help each other - you and Granny and Grandad and me - and Daddy when he has time.' He felt like an afterthought. 'We'll have to work hard and you mustn't mind if we can't play with you like we used to. And sometimes I expect we'll be extra tired and we might get cross - but it's only because there will be so much more to do. But we can do it.'

Through the chink in the door he saw her shifting her position on the cushions, dropping kisses on the child's sleeping head.

'One day I'll explain it all to you. How the doctors thought maybe our little baby - our Peter - might be better off dead. Dead indeed! When we are here to love him. That's why God chose our little family for this special baby. Because we've got so much love to give him. And because we know there are so many things that are much more important than being brainy. We aren't going to murder a tiny little baby. Certainly not! Specially our own little baby. What kind of monsters would we be if we did that - just because he isn't quite like other babies. Well, he isn't - he's special. He's specially special. And he's ours. We'll make him so happy, Victoria. Give him a specially happy life - to make up for all those horrid thoughts. And Granny - she'll help us.'

Richard felt a sudden flooding sensation go over him - like a wave of nausea. But he leaned against the wall, keeping his eyes on the tableau formed by his wife and daughter. Listening in spite of the silent screams within.

'So don't be unhappy, sweetheart - Mummy loves you every bit as much as she always did. But now you have to share me with Peter. And right now he needs me most. I have to give him all of my strength. Help him to win his battles so we can bring him home and be a real family again.'

With that she rose, holding the limp form close to her as she moved across to lay her on the bed. Gently, tenderly she covered Victoria with the patchwork cover she had so loved as a child herself. She knelt, caressing the flushed cheek, removing the last trace of the violent tears with a soft finger.

Fearing discovery and his own tense emotions, Richard shot into the bathroom where he stood with clenched fists and gritted teeth struggling with his own inner turmoil. So he was as good as a murderer, a monster, was he? Because he wanted what was best for her - peace, freedom from a lifelong burden.

He felt a coldness wash over him now as he recalled that struggle. Something in him had changed in that ten minutes before he faced Sue again. He couldn't quite comprehend what it was - but something was different because of that overhead revelation.

The following day they rang the hospital to see if it was possible to set up a meeting with one or more of the doctors. Told of their request, Roger instantly set aside a block of time that afternoon before going in search of Catherine. She had been deputed to seek out the opinions of her nursing colleagues. He needed to know if there was any cause for concern there. The right opportunity might be now. To get a decision made.

Roger found Catherine quietly feeding one of the infants who had survived months of intensive care and was now simply being fattened up in readiness for going home. She loved those moments when she could enjoy the rhythmic sucking, inwardly revel in the miracle she had helped to bring about. Two other nurses were also feeding well babies nearby. Roger knew he could not discuss such a sensitive subject with anyone else within earshot. He strolled up to the cotside and bent to caress with one finger the downy cheek of the premature infant, eyes tightly closed, every effort given to coordinating breathing and sucking.

'You're doing well, little man!' he murmured.

'Yes, he's finally got the hang of eating. But he's still playing up for his poor Mum, aren't you, Rory?'

'Don't you want to go home then?'

The baby's face was suddenly screwed up in a heavy frown and the sucking stopped. They both laughed at the infant's apparent response.

'When you've finished feeding Rory - can I have a moment of your time? I need you to bring me up to date - about the Flanaghan situation.'

'Certainly. I can come now if it would suit you better - rather than hanging around. I could get someone else to finish off this feed.'

'No, please. I've got plenty of work to get on with. A few more minutes won't make much difference. It's just that - the parents have asked to see me this afternoon. I'd like to know how everyone feels about the situation. In case this is the moment for decision-making.'

'Oh, I see. I should only be about ten more minutes.'

When Catherine appeared in his doorway, Roger rose to usher her in and close the door before speaking. Catherine sat forward in her seat at first, tense, not quite at ease.

'Have you had a chance to talk to your nurses - about Peter, I mean?' Roger's tone was quietly enquiring.

'Yes, I've talked to everyone who's been involved to any extent with him. Including the night staff,' she added.

'And what's your impression of the feeling - in general.'

'In general? Most of them feel happy to go along with whatever you and the parents feel is best. They don't have strong feelings either way. Most are relieved they don't have to make the decision!' she smiled rather wryly at him.

'And in particular?'

'There are three who feel quite strongly, I'd say. From that team meeting you'll know about Wendy Greenaway and Jo Manson. They're two of them. Wendy feels very strongly indeed that all life is sacred and not "disposable", as she phrases it. As you know, she's close to the family. She's keen to go on being supportive. But she's adamant that she won't have anything to do with withdrawing treatment. She says she'll have to refuse to be involved any further if the decision is to disconnect the ventilator.'

'And is your sense that - she might report such an action?'

'No, I really don't think she would. She's a good friend of mine - perhaps I should tell you that. I like her a lot. She's no shirker.'

'Oh I know that. I've been very impressed by her. She's an exceptionally good nurse.'

'Yes. She is. She's also very conscious of the weight of responsibility you carry. She was emphatic that she doesn't have a personal quarrel with you. You're entitled to your beliefs - as far as she's concerned. She respects that. She said she knows you really care for these families. But perhaps you don't know - she had a horrid experience - in another hospital - before she came here. She fell foul of one of her medical colleagues - somebody who was very unsympathetic to her beliefs - you know - gave her a hard time.'

'Hard that.'

'Yes. It's made her wary. But she has these very strong views and says she can't be untrue to what she thinks.'

'Absolutely. I understand that.'

'She knows you wouldn't give her a hard time. But she feels badly about what it might mean. Actually, she did say, it had been tremendously helpful to her to have an opportunity to say how she felt in a public forum - at the team meeting. She really appreciated being consulted - at this stage, you know - before the decision is finally made. Seemed to think it was really important.'

'Good. I presume if it came to it you could manage to use her effectively elsewhere - draft in someone else?'

'Oh yes. We can just reshuffle everyone. I should be sorry though. She's been great with those parents from the outset.'

'Would she want to explain to them herself - why she was withdrawing?'

'I think she would. She did say they knew how she felt about the sanctitiy of life so it wouldn't really surprise them.'

'What if the parents still wanted to talk with her and so on? If she wasn't involved in the physical care of the baby - could she take that on board?'

'Well, I must admit I didn't ask her that. I sort of assumed that she wouldn't want to. Well, it'd all be so difficult - being loyal - but supportive - when something was going on which her conscience told her was so morally wrong. Wouldn't it? I'd have preferred to keep her well out of all of it - myself.'

'OK. I see your point. So, is there someone else who could inherit her mantle with Sue and Richard, d'you think?'

'Oh, I think so. Eileen Shorten - she's super with them. And well - I'd be prepared to make myself more available for this last lap. If it comes to that. If you think ...'

'Of course. You'd be fine. What about during the night? Is there someone close enough to them there?'

'Yes. There's Bridget Doig and there's Rosamund Jeffery - you know them. Both very experienced sisters. They both know the family well. They don't have a problem with stopping treatment. One or other of them will be on every night.'

'OK. So we're covered that way. What about the other people with strong views. The student? Jo? Yes?'

'Jo Manson, yes.'

'She still leaning the other way?'

'Yes, she is. Emphatically!'

'Understandable. I actually met her in the corridor a couple of days after that meeting. Talked with her about her feelings on this matter - expressly. She was quite vociferous again.'

'So she told you - about her sister's circumstances.'

'Yes. You can see why she feels so strongly. I understand it. From all accounts the boy's three people's work.'

'Exactly. I think, reading between the lines, it sounds like it's a question of lack of support and services as much as anything. I think. But anyway she isn't, personally, going to have a problem with any decision made about Peter. We'll just keep her and Wendy apart for a bit I think! Wendy was certainly pretty upset - Jo had a go at her after the meeting on Monday. She was really upset.'

'Oh, dear. That's a pity. Pity when it gets personal. Makes it harder.'

'It would be perfectly natural for me to have only senior staff in with Peter - for the last bit anyway. So I wouldn't be involving Jo in his care. I must admit I wasn't keen to involve her - you remember - she offered. Did she say any more to you, about talking to the parents?'

'We did mention it in passing. I simply said if it seemed appropriate I'd let her know, but in the meantime it was probably best if she didn't raise the matter with them - or at least not until we have a clearer idea of how they will jump. I think she followed the argument. I told her that I thought it would be an added burden - having someone tell you how horrendous it will be - if you've decided that you're going to take the kiddie home.'

'Oh, I'm glad you cleared that. I wasn't sure how to answer her. I was a bit afraid - well, perhaps it was my personal resistance. Well, she is a bit - abrasive - at times. I didn't want to crush her offer - but I can't help feeling she's a bit too prejudiced to be able to keep the discussion balanced. And I also wonder - p'rhaps she isn't the right person for Sue and Richard. They seem so gentle and quiet. She could be too dominating for them. But that's just my personal feeling. Not that she isn't a great nurse. And of course she might be quite different on her own with the parents.' Her hasty qualifier made him smile.

'I know. But I know too what you mean about her manner. And I agree. I wouldn't choose her for these parents. But we can probably arrange things so she doesn't feel rejected.'

'There's one other person I'm not so sure about. That's Sally Oswald. She's a part-time person. Staff nurse on night duty. Does two nights a week. It wasn't so much what she said, as the probing. I had an uneasy feeling about her questions. She's been here about four years and I don't know - I don't have any evidence - not that she's blown the whistle or anything. But there was something. I think we should be careful about her.'

'Would you like me to talk with her?' Roger raised his eyebrows in enquiry.

'Well, thanks - but I don't think so - at least not yet. If you singled her out it might look as if I was suspicious. I'll try to have another talk with her if the decision is to stop treatment - see if she wants to have a chance to discuss things with you - if that's all right with you?'

Roger nodded, content to leave it to her good judgement.

'My medical colleagues don't present a problem. Bill Forsyth's examined Peter carefully and agrees with my prognosis.'

'And what time are you seeing the parents?'

Roger glanced at his watch.

'In exactly three quarters of a hour.'

'Well, good luck. Shall I arrange for a tray of tea?'

'That would be a kindness, thanks,' he smiled gratefully. It helped to have the support of these experienced people who felt the pain with him. They knew what it cost to agonise over these cases. He was not alone.

Even so he felt alone as he closed the door of the Quiet Room and poured tea for Sue and Richard Flanaghan. They all settled back into the great armchairs but each knew the physical comfort did not reflect a mental ease.

'You wanted to see me?' Roger opened the discussion gently to give them space to inch their way into the difficult bits at their own pace.

'Yes. We know - you've been considering whether to continue with Peter's treatment or not.' Richard swallowed hard. This was not easy in spite of his rehearsal. So much hung on these questions. He felt in some way responsible for the answers he would get. Important to phrase it right. 'I suppose we want more information. About the damage - what it means in real terms.'

That stalled for time a bit. Going over the 'facts'.

'Well, as you know, it's impossible to talk in absolute certainties, here. We can only give you what we think is the case - from our experience with other babies - the results of Peter's tests - about what lies ahead for him. You understand?'

Both parents nodded. There was a curious tension in the air. Like before a thunderstorm. Roger couldn't precisely define it but he felt its effect. He decided to change tack.

'I actually think it would be helpful, in the first instance, if you could tell me what you understand to be the position as far as Peter is concerned. Could we start there?'

Richard turned to Sue.

'D'you want to start off?'

She shook her head vigorously and Roger knew from her clenched hand on the cup that she was struggling with her control. He gave her a half smile.

Richard's voice was deliberately clipped as he recounted the 'facts'.

'As I understand it - he's suffered brain damage. You think its severe enough to mean he'll be partially paralysed, mentally impaired, possibly - probably - blind. You don't think he'll ever be capable of independent existence. And his lungs - they're damaged too. He's unlikely to be weaned off of oxygen for a long time yet. He'll be very vulnerable to infections - probably for years. There's a good chance he won't see his tenth birthday. But on the other hand, with modern medication - good care - there's also a chance that he could outlive both of us.'

Roger felt a vague disquiet at the tenor of Richard's catalogue. His face was inscrutible. He sat perfectly still fingers loosely holding his cup and saucer and as soon as he had completed his speech he took a sip of the hot tea with a steady hand. What was behind this calm recital?

The doctor turned to Sue. Much as he wanted to protect her, he knew he could do little to soften this traumatic experience except be kindly in the delivery of his blows.

'Could you ...?' he gently encouraged her.

'You can't be sure of any of that. It's only what you think is likely. He could go on - prove everybody wrong. You said yourself - sometimes they surprise everyone. I know you don't think it's likely. But - but I want to go on hoping. Maybe - maybe there'll be - a miracle. And even if there isn't a miracle - well, as long as he knows how much he's loved and wanted. And he is.'

There was a long silence as she finished abruptly, a caught breath adding to the poignancy of her words. Pain gripped Roger's heart as he thanked her. He had to dent this bubble.

'You're right. We can't be certain. But we are more certain in Peter's case than in lots of cases. I must be honest with you. He's had a massive bleed into his head. His lungs are in very bad shape indeed. We are concerned - very concerned - not to have him suffer pain. As you know, we've been giving him a little morphine so that it doesn't hurt him every time the ventilator shoots air into his lungs. I suppose what we have to look at is this. At what point, if any, does Peter's prognosis - his future outlook - become so poor that it's unacceptable - morally unacceptable to prolong his life?'

'So is this about his pain - **his** suffering? Not ours?' Richard's voice was taut.

'Yes, at the moment, anyway. We have to ask ourselves, I think - when do the burdens of continuing to exist - in this way - outweigh the benefits of just being alive? For Peter.'

'But you can't say he'd rather be dead than alive! I mean, he doesn't know. He doesn't know what life's about.' Sue's face struggled between bewilderment and conviction.

'No, and that's part of the dilemma. Because he can't tell us how he feels. So **we** have to decide for him when enough is enough.' Roger looked from one to the other.

'Yes, that's right. He doesn't know. But we know. We all know what real pain's like. We know whether we'd want to be blind - incontinent - unable to feed ourselves and walk and talk - unable to relate to other people. We know what we'd want - if we were like that - if we'd want to be left to suffer or put out of our misery.' Richard's voice had a hard edge which made Roger watch him more carefully. 'We've got to think about what it's like for him, darling.'

Sue had shrunk in on herself and sat staring miserably into her cup twisting her finger in and around the handle. Eventually she raised her glistening eyes and asked Roger a direct question.

'D'you think - you can - you are controlling the pain? So he isn't suffering.'

'Well, it's difficult to be sure. We're trying and we think we have it under control - but of course he can't tell us it's OK. We can only go by the signs he gives us and the machine readings.'

'But you feel pretty sure - he's not in any pain?'

'As far as I can tell he's not - at the moment anyway.'

'And will you be able to keep it like that - keep him free from pain - as he grows up?'

'I couldn't guarantee that - not that he'd never be in any pain. I wouldn't always be looking after him anyway. But I suppose - well, most of us do suffer pain - at some points in our lives - don't we.'

'So he wouldn't suffer more than we all do?' Sue was persisting. Roger felt uneasy. He didn't want to be forced into a corner. There were too many imponderables.

'I can't say. It all depends - how he progresses - just what's wrong with him.'

'But it's always uncertain anyway. So - that shouldn't make us decide he's better ... dead.' Her voice crumbled over the word. She shivered slightly, regained her composure and turning to her husband, laid a hand on his knee as she spoke.

'So, Richard. He's not suffering. That's good, isn't it? And there's never any promise in life that it'll be easy. So - he'll just take his chance with the rest of us. OK - with a few more problems perhaps but ...'

Temporarily free from their searching glances, Roger had leisure to watch them closely. He felt again the uneasy feeling that something was discordant here. But he couldn't put a finger on what it was. They were simply presenting two sides of an argument in an effort to arrive at the most momentous decision of their lives.

Richard laid a reassuring hand over his wife's and nodded. 'OK. But what about the work load for you?'

'That's irrelevant. We couldn't ... kill,' she shot the word out, 'Kill our baby just because it was a lot of work for us.'

'If I may,' Roger's interjection was at once apologetic but commanding. 'I think - no matter how distasteful it seems at the moment - and I accept that it's difficult - you must consider what you're taking on. Oh, I know it's hard - it's hard to think of yourselves when we're actually considering whether Peter lives or not. But your welfare's important too. This will put an enormous strain on you both - make no mistake about that. It will. Only you can decide how much you can take. But - it will strain your health, your sense of well-being, your marriage. There's a strong possibility that you'll lose him at some point anyway - even if we do pull out all the stops now. I think you have to consider whether you're prepared to risk these other things - for what? - an outside chance of him ever knowing you or returning your love?' They would never know how much it hurt him to utter those words. He had himself after all risked all and Ginny had come out of it more devoted to him than ever. But Ginny was Ginny.

But to Richard three words cut deep - 'strain ... your marriage.'

'My only concern is for you, darling.' He gripped her hand so hard she winced.

'I know, dear. But I know we can do it - we can be strong for each other. And after all - we don't do this for any reward. Even if he doesn't know us, it'll be enough that we love him. And you never know - maybe he'll surprise us all - in time. Maybe he'll get to know us - that would just be a bonus.'

Something in his face seemed to bring her back from her distant imagery. 'Richard, you do think - you do agree - it's right to keep on trying? Oh, say you do! To please me, tell me you agree!'

'If that's what you want - if you're sure you can cope - OK, so be it.' His words soothed her and she turned back to Roger with a calm expression. Roger, himself, was anything but reassured however. He continued to discuss the details of the practical management of the baby as if the matter was settled. Inwardly he resolved that he must speak with Richard alone. Sue's position was quite clear. But that had been too easy an acquiescence. It was there again - that sense that something was not what it seemed.

His moment came unexpectedly when Sue rather embarrassed excused herself to go to the lavatory. Seizing the brief opportunity, Roger launched without preamble.

'I get the impression you aren't as sure as your wife, Richard.'

Richard looked startled.

'Do you want us to continue treating Peter?' The question sounded so harsh. No time to wrap it up.

'Well, I am worried about Sue coping - the burden on her - years of it. Yes, you're right I am concerned. But you see how sure she is - sure she can do it. I can't seem to doubt her ability. If that's what she wants ...' He shrugged his shoulders.

Roger noticed he avoided eye contact. His body language, his tone - it disturbed him. Vaguely. Nothing he could pinpoint.

'Maybe we should have another discussion a bit further down the line,' he was tentative.

'No!' The response was emphatic, decisive. 'No more. It won't make any difference. It'll only upset Sue - if you keep raising it. Look, I know her. She's been consistent from the outset. She can't bear to think of him - dying. And I don't want her upset any more. It's my fault we had this meeting today - it's only because I wasn't ready to make the commitment. Make a definite decision. Don't think I don't know - I do. I know what it'll cost her. But if that's what she wants ... That's the end of the matter. No point in going over and over it.' Richard rose to his feet abruptly. He held out his hand to Roger. 'Thank you for all your help. I know you meant well, telling us about the problems. And you've been very kind. Thanks for everything.'

The handshake seemed to seal something but Roger was unsure what. He knew without doubt that the conversation had been closed. He was left with an uncomfortable feeling. It was incomplete. He hadn't said so much he wanted to say. He felt out-manouevred in some strange unsettling way.

But his farewells to these parents were warm as he assured them of as much continuing support as they needed. They left, Richard's arm protectively around his wife as they walked past the nursery to the lift on their way home. Roger was left - reliving the past hour. Peter was left - battling for every breath.

CHAPTER 9

Out of Our Hands

It was evening time. Wendy luxuriated in the peace around her. She was in charge of Peter tonight and as the Unit was not too busy he had her undivided attention. Being a perfectionist she liked nothing better than to be able to concentrate on one baby. She had, too, an inner peace. It had been such a relief to hear that the parents had opted to have treatment continue. She didn't want to have to desert them in their hour of need. This meant she could be around to support them and prepare them for the time ahead when they must care for this damaged child on their own. Deep inside she felt a strong desire to pass on some of her own conviction that they were entrusted with a very precious charge.

The rhythmic swish of the ventilator, the hum of the incubator and the slight hissing of the oxygen were familiar sounds and she was undisturbed by them as she read a document on infection control which had recently been circulated to all departments. Peter needed only half-hourly observations so she was using the intervals to catch up on the literature. But the words kept blurring. Even second - third reading - she didn't take it in. The events of the past few days had disturbed her deeply. She couldn't seem to obliterate the memories.

She heard again the strident tones of Jo in the changing room - sneering - so unpleasant. The sick feeling came again - just thinking about it - remembering. It was just the kind of encounter she hated. Such a long way from the gentleness, the understanding of Mother Maria - the other nuns. Oh that was what it ought to be like - like St Agnes - the nuns - the peace, the caring. Maybe she was in the wrong place.

It had been hard - exposing her views to public scrutiny at the Unit meeting. It took courage. And then to get Jo's abrasive response - in front of everybody - it was not easy staying cool. But she had to hang on to her dignity. Not sink to the personal attack - Jo's level. And she'd learned from the nuns - important not to let it cloud your judgement - stop you caring yourself.

Stop her caring about Jo - about her nephew - her sister. That's why she'd gone out of her way to offer the suggestion of a new assessment for Greg - in spite of the hostility.

She'd seen the effect of years of sorrow on families. Over and over again. If anything could possibly alleviate their suffering - wasn't it worth a try? But what did she get? 'Cranky ideas' ... 'people poking their noses in'... 'too cruel' ... 'took you three years - three years and you got out.' What a cheek! She hadn't 'got out'. It was time to move on. But she still cared - understood - returned when she could. Instead of taking a holiday - jetting off into the sun - she went to St Agnes to help out. Jo hadn't really heard that - didn't want to. Bent on being aggressive. Would probably sneer at that too anyway.

Best to concentrate on the good she could do - not dwell on the negative experiences. Easy to get things out of perspective. Especially easy when you were emotionally stressed. Peter - he needed her. Sue and Richard - they didn't seem to think she was a crank - interfering. She could help them. And now she didn't have to desert them. Things weren't all bad.

Frequent glances at Peter reassured her that he was peaceful at the moment. Recordings were stable and he seemed restful. He had even started to tolerate small amounts of milk down his nasogastric tube better. As she gently percussed the boney rib cage to loosen the secretions, she talked softly to him telling him about the experiences of life ahead for him. And when all the invasive procedures were completed she stood circling his fragile frame in her hands - protecting, giving a sense of containment, of security. Gradually his heart rate decreased, his brow unfurrowed. Not until he had fully relaxed and recovered his stability did she withdraw her protection and resume her reading. So often it was necessary to immediately turn to another baby equally in need of intensive care and these extra touches - the refinements - the art of caring - had to be shelved. It pleased her to be able to mix the art with the science. He responded well to such management.

The time passed slowly until Catherine came to relieve her for a meal break. She was careful to complete a full set of observations before leaving. This left Catherine free to work on off-duty rosters as she sat beside Peter for that short half-hour. When Wendy returned she was surprised to see Richard in the room. She smiled warmly at him.

'Late visit tonight. Peter will be surprised to feel your touch again today - but I'm sure he'll be pleased.'

Richard's only response was a rather tight smile and a shrug. His glance darted from Catherine to Wendy unsure about the mechanics of what came next.

'Richard was asking when you'd be back. He knew you were on tonight,' Catherine said, rising from the stool and folding her papers together.

'Peter's been a good boy in your absence. No change in anything since you left. But I notice you are almost out of 20ml syringes and I'll bring you some more distilled water.'

'Oh, I actually have more syringes but I put them in the cupboard over there to save cluttering things up nearby. But thanks, it would be helpful to have the water ready,' Wendy smiled at her colleague. These two women both liked and respected each other and were enjoying the rare opportunity to work together.

When Catherine had left, Richard moved in closer to the incubator.

'How's he seem tonight?'

'Grand. He's really restful and nice and stable.'

'So, there's no chance of him ... you know ... not tonight?'

'Dying, d'you mean?'

Richard nodded, eyes on his son.

'I wouldn't think so. Not unless something dramatic happens. He's holding his own quite nicely, aren't you, little fellow?' Her voice dropped to a caress as she too looked at the fledgling boy.

'He seems very still.'

'Yes, he's sleeping between treatments. Nice when he seems contented, isn't it?'

'Yep. I hate it when he thrashes around in there - his face all screwed up - purple. Looks like he's yelling - but there's no sound - horrible. I hate it. He seems so ... I don't know ... angry? hurt?'

'I know what you mean. But he's great tonight. Nice that you can enjoy this peaceful time with him, eh?'

Richard was staring unblinkingly at Peter as if in deep thought but a brief nod indicated he had heard. Wendy moved aside and gestured to him to come closer to the incubator. She moved her stool away and settled herself with her reading in the corner of the room, leaving father and son in a private world for a few precious minutes.

'Will it disturb him - if I touch him?' Richard spoke in a whisper.

'Not if you just hold his hand or stroke his skin gently. Something pleasant. Please do - just go ahead. Ignore me.'

Richard's touch was wonderingly tentative at first. But then, finding the baby remained curled and unruffled, he ventured a firmer movement on the downy skin.

After ten minutes, Wendy was reluctant to disturb them but observations had to be made. She explained her intention and Richard moved to stand staring out of the window as she performed the necessary tasks.

As she worked she apologised for the intrusion.

'It's OK. I understand.'

But Wendy was still uneasy. He seemed somehow upset by the interruption - distant, distracted. Suddenly he spoke, still without turning.

'I was wondering. Would it be possible - OK - for me to be with him - on my own? You know, without anyone else in the room?'

Wendy understood the discomfort of other eyes always watching parents as they related to their babies. It was like being in a goldfish bowl. She herself intensely disliked everyone watching her work when the medical rounds were in progress. It made her less nimble, somehow, more self-conscious about the things she normally did so deftly.

'I don't see why not. I'm afraid it would only be for about a quarter of an hour. Is that OK?'

Richard nodded, expressionless.

'There's usually nothing needing to be done between the half-hour readings. He should be fine. But if there's anything - don't hesitate. Ring the emergency buzzer - if you're anxious in any way. I can be here in seconds.'

Without looking at her, Richard answered, 'Thanks.'

Wendy waited until Peter was quite settled and then smiled warmly again as she beckoned him closer.

'All yours then.'

They both stood for a long quiet moment looking down at the sleeping form.

'Don't hesitate - ring if you need me.'

With the words she slipped out. Good chance to get a coffee and have a brief chat with Catherine. The senior sister was surprised to see her but nodded her agreement with Wendy's decision. Peter was unusually stable tonight. And the parents had been through the mill today.

'It's almost as if Peter knows his future is safe now. He's lovely and peaceful tonight,' Wendy mused.

'Good. It'll help Richard to see him looking so contented. He was really pleased that you were looking after Peter. You've obviously made a big impression on them.'

'That was kind - but they're a really nice couple. Oh, I do hope things work out for them. They've had rotten luck.'

They sat companionably sipping coffee and exchanging occasional comments, Wendy keeping a watchful eye on the clock even as she enjoyed the unscheduled break. Even when the stated time was up she stretched expansively, reluctant to intrude into this fragile family scene. But she knew Richard understood really.

Re-entering the room she was surprised to see no sign of him leaning over the incubator. Odd. You'd have expected him to stay till she returned. But at least she needn't feel guilty about breaking into their private space. She moved straight to the incubator to prepare the equipment for the next dose of physiotherapy and suction. Simultaneously opening her mouth to speak to the baby and reaching for the catheters, she recoiled in shocked disbelief.

Peter lay flat on his back, the ventilator tube disconnected and the intravenous line dangling free in the air. She was suddenly aware of the silence - no swish or hiss mingled with the hum. Both ventilator and oxygen were switched off. The monitor was without a trace. Switched off too. Only the incubator hummed. No respiratory effort. No heartbeat.

In an instant Wendy had leapt to press the emergency bell. Flinging open the whole side of the incubator she blasted oxygen into the face of the infant as she compressed his chest vigorously. One. Two. Three. Four. The sound of running feet. Five. Pause. One. Two. Three. Catherine was beside her.

'What happened?'

'Get a bag and mask, quickly! He's not breathing!'

More running feet.

'Get a doctor - quickly!'

Wendy kept pumping.

'What happened?'

What had happened? She couldn't think about that. There was a life at stake here. Time for questions later.

Other hands passed tubes, filled syringes, held masks, injected drugs. Her fingers stayed on the little chest. Pumping. Pumping. Pumping. Counting silently. Willing him to breathe. Willing the heart to start beating again.

Roger's voice now, calm, commanding. Telling her gently to stop. She couldn't stop. His voice again, compelling, strong. Stop! Peter's life depended on her. Pump. Pump. Pump. Roger now physically removing her. Didn't he understand? Peter needed her. Roger's hand not hers on the stethoscope now on that chest wall. His fingers lifting the eyelids, closing them - finally, lingering on the cheek.

'I'm sorry. He's gone.'

He couldn't be. He was stable. She was in charge of him. Wendy stared wild-eyed at the still, purplish form on the crumpled white sheet. The remnants of their struggle littered the surfaces cluttering the area all around Peter's body - untidy, uncared for.

Dimly she heard Roger ushering people out of the room, felt Catherine's arm around her shoulders coaxing her into the low seat. Her eyes remained transfixed on the baby. He **couldn't** be dead! It didn't make sense.

A hot mug of strong tea was in her hands. Trembling hands. She choked on it. Catherine's arm around her. Silent support. Everyone waiting.

Silently waiting. What for? For her to drink that tea. She hated tea. It tasted bitter. Far too strong. Couldn't stop shivering. What was the matter with her? Blanket round her - like a road accident. Tea all gone. Hands took the empty mug.

Roger drew up a low chair beside hers. What kind eyes he has she thought detachedly. No smile now though.

'Wendy, I know you've had a dreadful shock but I need to know - what happened. What happened here tonight?'

Her voice sounded mechanical, detached, remote.

'Peter was fine - really stable. Tolerating his feeds well. After each observation - I held him with my hands - you know - like this,' she cupped her hands around the imaginery baby, 'Until he settled and went to sleep. He likes that, you know, being held still.'

Roger's gaze remained steady. His nod understood.

'Everything was fine. And Richard came. Really nice - nice for him to see Peter - relaxed, peaceful. Not fighting. He liked being here without Sue -

having Peter to himself. He reached in and stroked him - ever so gently. Didn't want to disturb Peter's sleep. Lovely to see them together like that. Real father and son.'

'And then?'

'I had to break the spell. The observations were due. Richard didn't like it - seemed unhappy. Said he understood - but he didn't like it.'

'How could you tell that?'

'He was tense. Didn't smile. Kept his back to me.'

'And then what happened?'

'Then he asked me - would it be possible for him to be really on his own with Peter. I knew what he meant. It's not the same when there's somebody else in the room. Peter was really good. Really stable. Relaxed. Better than he's ever been. Richard's really gentle with him. I said it would be OK. If he was anxious - just to ring the emergency bell.' The words were flowing more easily now. That tea had thawed her frozen mind.

'I finished the observations for seven and then left him with Peter. I went to get a coffee and had a chat with Catherine. When I came back in ...'

'What time was that?' He sounded like a policeman.

'Twenty five past.'

'Seven?'

'Yes.'

'So you left him alone with Peter for twenty minutes at the most?'

'Not even that. By the time I'd finished the seven o'clock obs and cleared up and filled in the charts it was after ten past.'

'So it was just over fifteen minutes they were left alone.'

'Yes. Just over fifteen minutes.'

'And when you came back into the room?'

'I was surprised. He wasn't here. I expected to see him leaning over the incubator stroking Peter. But no - no sign of him.'

Great quivering intakes of breath began to punctuate her words.

'Peter was lying on his back ... dreadful colour - purplish ... The ET tube was ... out ... lying on the sheet ... The monitors ... the ventilator ... the oxygen ... all switched off.'

Catherine's arm again, comforting.

'I pressed the bell ... started resuscitating. Then Catherine came ... and the others.' Her voice faded away and she dropped her head into her hands.

The wracking gasps were harder to hear than weeping.

'What have I ... done? Oh, ... what have ... I done?'

Roger's tone was gentle.

'You mustn't blame yourself. I think under the circumstances we'd probably all have done the same thing. You couldn't have known he had this in mind.'

'It must have been Richard ...' Even as she uttered the words she disbelieved them.

'I'm afraid it looks like it.'

'How could he ...? How could he? His own little baby!' It was beyond her imagining.

'We won't know that until we talk to him. At the moment we don't know where he is. But Sue has to be told.'

She raised stricken eyes to his. The dawning horror in her face appalled Roger and Catherine. Roger touched her arm briefly.

'No need for you to see her.'

'I must. I was looking after Peter.'

'You really don't have to. I'll see her.'

'Have you told her?'

'Not yet. First I must phone the police and ask them how we should proceed. I imagine they will want to speak to Richard first but I need to know at what point I can speak to Sue - how much we can disclose.'

'Poor, poor woman,' Wendy shuddered. 'How will she ever understand this?'

How could he ever tell her, Roger agonised.

Inspector Crammond was calm and business like. He listened attentively to Roger's account.

'I'll send a couple of men around. Just leave everything just as it is, sir. Don't let anyone in and keep everybody there who's been on duty this evening. And don't let anyone touch anything.'

'Well, we've had to touch things. Had to try to resuscitate the baby.'

'Pity about that. Suppose you had to though, I see your point there. Oh, well, don't do anything else until my chaps arrive. They'll be as quick as they can be.'

'What about telling the mother?'

'Best wait until we have a better idea of what's going on.'

'And if she phones?'

'Stall for time sir. We'll be as quick as we can.'

'And what about the father?'

'We'll attend to that side of things, sir. Can you give me a description of the man? - what sort of car he drives? - anything else that might help us find him?'

Roger replied almost mechanically, his thoughts racing ahead to the moment when he must tell Sue Flanaghan her little boy was dead. At the hands of his father.

Sergeant Jeffery Littlestone and WPC Celia Thomas arrived within ten minutes of his call. Roger forestalled them in the corridor requesting extreme care in dealing with Sister Greenaway. She was a particularly sensitive and compassionate nurse. Very close to this family. This experience had been extremely traumatic for her. She didn't need to be made to feel like a criminal.

'We'll be careful, sir. But thanks for the warning. Helps to know what we're dealing with. Can we see the scene of the crime first?'

Both officers looked with pity on the tiny corpse spreadeagled inelegantly over the stained sheet.

'Never seen one that small before,' the sergeant's tone was muted.

The constable concentrated on scribbling facts into her notebook. It turned her stomach to look at this travesty of a human being. She had always found it hard going dealing with the bodies she had to inspect in her job - this one was particularly upsetting. Their questions related to logistics and organization as they struggled to understand the workings of this rarified world. Roger could only take them so far. The real details would come from the person who had been responsible for little Peter Flanaghan tonight - Wendy Greenaway.

Wendy repeated her story in a flat, dispassionate tone cradling herself in her arms and staring blankly ahead as if focusing on this once familiar room would be too much for her composure. Her Welsh accent was more than usually pronounced. As if she had given up on control. Even gentle probing seemed to question her competence and both Roger and Catherine kept anxious eyes on the huddled form. She had requested that they stay but they felt unsure of what was permissible in terms of support. Interrogation of a colleague wasn't part of the normal experience. When the two custodians of the law had satisfied themselves that they understood what had happened in general rather than medical terms, they rose to their feet and replaced their notebooks with grave faces.

'The mother'll have to be told.'

'Would it be permissible for me to come with you - help with breaking the news?' Roger's voice was tentative. There were unfamiliar boundaries here.

'Probably be a good thing. Less of a shock initially if she sees someone she knows. But one of us'll have to accompany you I'm afraid, sir.'

'Yes, of course. I understand. OK if we tidy up the baby - make him more presentable - before his mother sees him?'

'Yes, we've finished here now. Not much evidence when everything's been disturbed since the act anyway.'

A raised eyebrow in Catherine's direction left matters in her hands and Roger followed the policemen to the door. On an impulse he turned back and walked over to the crumpled figure in the chair. Crouching down beside her chair he spoke gently.

'Wendy, I'm going out to see Sue now. I expect she'll want to come back in to see Peter. Do you want to go home or to stay here or what? There is absolutely no need for you to see the family just yet. Catherine and I can deal with that side of things.'

The staring blankness of her eyes told its own tale but she was insistent that she help prepare the baby's body and be there to say something to Sue if she returned to the hospital.

'OK. If you're sure. But if you change your mind when the moment comes, no-one will think any the worse of you. You've had an appalling shock. And we know how close you've been to this family.'

'That's why I have to do this - for Peter - for Sue.'

It was a strange experience sitting beside the stolid figure in navy uniform driving through the streets in a marked car. Had he not been so tense about the coming encounter, Roger might even have enjoyed the feeling of other-worldness. But a sick feeling in his stomach was more than travel queasiness.

He made sure he was standing in first line of vision at the door as the Sergeant rang the bell. Through the glass panel at eye level he saw the light shining on bouncing fair hair and knew it would be Sue not Richard who would open the door to this unlikely combination of callers. He noted with relief that the policeman had moved to one side as she approached. He'd be out of her sight - initially - temporarily.

'Why, Dr Carshalton! What a surprise. Do come in.' Although surprised, her instinctive reaction was to accord him the welcome she gave to any acquaintance visiting her home. It was something in his slow movement forward and his demeanour that first rang alarm bells. He wasn't his usual calm, confident self.

'Something wrong? Is it - Peter?' Cold fingers clutched at her heart.

'I'm afraid so.'

Even as Roger's words dropped into the suspended moment, her eyes darted behind him to the policeman. She recoiled bewildered, suddenly fearful - fearful of something unknown - terrible.

'Is Richard home?' Roger schooled himself to ask the question in an ordinary tone.

'No - he's not back yet. He came in to the hospital to see Peter. Oh, what is it? Has there been ...? Is he ... is he dead? ' The voice sank to a hoarse whisper. She had both hands clutching her face, eyes wide, as she backed into the living room followed by the two men.

'Please, Sue, sit down. I'm afraid - you've guessed - it's bad news.' Roger helped her down and sat beside her on the sofa.

'Is it ...? Peter ... Is he worse?'

'I'm so very, very sorry, Sue. I'm afraid it is Peter. He died a little while ago.'

'Oh, no, no, no,' her voice pleaded with him to deny it.

He shook his head sadly giving her space for a moment before he had to tell her something even more devastating.

'What happened? They said - I thought they said - he was stable.'

'He was. But I'm afraid something rather awful happened tonight.'

She sat back from him, horrorstruck - unable to imagine what could have brought a policeman and a neonatologist to her home.

'As you know, Richard came in to see Peter tonight. He asked to be left alone with your little boy.'

'He was already dead - when Richard arrived?' Sue's voice rose almost accusingly in her mystification. Why hadn't they told her if it was so long ago?

'No. No. He was alive then. Richard wanted to spend time with him on his own. He asked the nurse to leave them alone. She thought he just wanted privacy. Peter was stable, restful - so she left them alone - for about a quarter of an hour.' Roger was finding it horrendously difficult to break this woman's heart. 'When the nurse went back into the room ... Peter was dead.'

'But how? What happened? Where's Richard? Peter died when he was alone with him! Oh, poor Richard. What a ghastly thing for him.'

Roger took a deep breath. He must do it or the policeman would have to. Better coming from him. She knew him at least.

'I'm afraid - Sue, I'm sorry - I'm terribly sorry - but it looks as if Richard did something - something to stop Peter breathing.'

Her look of utter incredulity seemed to destroy the trust between them at that moment.

'He wouldn't. Richard? He loved Peter as much as I did.'

'I know. We thought so too. In fact I still think - he did - he did love him deeply. We don't understand - quite why - why he did this. We'll have to wait until he can tell us. At the moment we can't - we don't know where he is. But the police are looking for him.'

'The police? The police are looking for Richard?'

'We just want to talk to him at the moment, ma'am. Hear what he has to say about this.' Sergeant Littlestone was distinctly uncomfortable. This traumatized woman was enduring more than any common criminal ever could. Life was a sod at times.

'Can I go and ... see Peter.' For the first time her voice broke.

'Yes, of course. We'll take you there. But first - can you bear it? - the Sergeant needs to ask you a few questions.'

'I'm really sorry, Mrs Flanaghan. We'll be as quick as we can. Just routine questions.' The sergeant took out his notebook and pen grateful for the excuse not to look at Sue. 'At what time did your husband leave the house?'

The questions seemed so unimportant. Sue's vague dismissive answers betrayed that her mind was elsewhere. Who cared about the timing of events, what Richard had said, how he had seemed. She hadn't really taken much notice. It was all so trivial. It wouldn't change the facts - Peter was dead.

'And did your husband seem in any way different this evening?'

'Different? I don't know. I don't think so. I didn't notice anything at the time. Well, perhaps ...'

'Yes?'

'Perhaps he - he hugged me - harder than sometimes when he said goodbye.' Sounded silly - personal - telling somebody else.

'And when he said goodbye can you remember - his exact words?'

'He didn't say much. Told me how much he loved me. But he often does that. What did he say? I don't think he actually said 'Goodbye' - more like 'Take care'. I didn't specially notice. Well, you don't - do you? But he always gave me a hug - kissed me if he was going anywhere - just in case - you know?'

'In case ...?'

'Sounds silly when you say it - but we always did - in case, you know - in case there was an accident - we didn't get the chance ...'

'I see. And it was just the same - today - like it normally was?'

'I think so - I didn't notice - anything different, I mean. Except - perhaps - maybe it was a closer hug - I don't know.'

'And you didn't suspect anything - anything out of the ordinary?'

Sue shook her head. Her bleak expression made the policeman want to put away his notebook and make her a cup of tea. Instead he gritted his teeth and persisted.

'Could you tell us where he might have gone - after - the hospital?'
'I've no idea. He must be terribly upset. But I don't know where he would go - except home.'

'When he has a worry of some kind normally, does he drive around, or go somewhere to think, or talk about it, or what?'

'He just goes very quiet - withdrawn. But otherwise he just carries on as normal.'

'What about parents? His still alive?'

'Yes, they live at Comptonfields. You know it? About 30 miles away.'

He nodded, scribbling in his pad. She gave the address mechanically.

'Any brothers or sisters - close friends he might go to?'

She rose to get the address book from beside the telephone. It felt odd giving such personal information to a complete stranger.

'We'll do our best, ma'am. But if you hear from him - if he comes back here - if someone else sees him - will you let us know, please?'

'Yes, of course. But I wanted - to go - to see Peter. He might return - while I'm away.'

'Oh, we'll be leaving one of our officers outside - just in case. It'll be quite all right for you to go to the hospital, ma'am. WPC Thomas is outside. Got the car. She'll run you and the doctor to the hospital. Is there anyone

- anyone you could call - someone who could stay with you - afterwards?'

Dully she answered. 'My mother. I'd better ring her - tell her.'

It was difficult dialling the familiar number, her fingers didn't seem like her own. The one-sided conversation sounded strained, unreal to the listening men.

'Mum, it's me ... Yes, I'm fine ... Oh that's good. Has she behaved today? ... Is she asleep? ... I was wondering, could you - could you leave her with Dad - come over. There's something - I want to talk to you about ... Thanks. I'd appreciate it ... See you in a few minutes then. Bye for now.'

Replacing the receiver, Sue looked at the two men, shaking her head slightly.

'Not on the phone. I didn't want to tell her - not over the phone. It'll be such a shock to her. I'll tell her - when she gets here.'

'Would you like one of us to tell her?' Roger asked cautiously.

'No, thanks. I'll do it. Just not over the phone - not when she has to drive here. Can I make you both a cup of tea while we wait?'

Her calm seemed unnatural but Roger had seen this form of numbness protecting people so often before. He accepted her offer. Better for her to be occupied. Simply sitting - that wouldn't help - trying to fight off the realization - Peter's catastrophic end - Richard's involvement. Telling her mother - that'd be hard - very hard indeed. It would start to sink in. Telling someone for the first time that her baby was dead - it would start to become a reality.

They toyed with the tea, no-one touching the plate of biscuits.

At the ring of the doorbell, Sue sat for a moment eyes closed as if in prayer before she rose unsteadily and went to greet her mother.

'Hello, darling. Came as soon as I could. But your Dad needed a hand holding the door he's rehanging - study door. Been rubbing the carpet for ages. He's got round to it at last. So I just stayed to help him. Bit of encouragement, you know. Didn't think a few minutes would make much difference. But here I am now.' Liz Mathieson had entered her daughter's home hundreds of times and there was nothing to alert her to the fact that there was anything different on this occasion from all the others. She hung her coat on the nearby hook and turned to smile at Sue.

'How are you, love? ...' Her voice trailed away as she met her daughter's eyes. 'Sue, what is it?'

'Oh Mum! It's Peter. He's ... he's dead.' She crumpled into her mother's outstretched arms and the tears flowed at last.

'Oh no. Oh, Sue, I'm so sorry. Oh, the poor little chap.'

She soothed and patted - dabbing at her own eyes with a rapidly disintegrating tissue. Gradually the facts emerged - the facts as Sue understood them. The aching grandmother found it so difficult to know what to say. Richard had been a model son-in-law. She and Harry had both welcomed him into their family - genuinely, warmly. He was such a gentle caring soul - so thoughtful and kind. Bit obsessive about Sue perhaps - but he'd made her so happy. And now they were saying he had ... murdered their grandson? There must be some mistake.

When the storm of acute distress had subsided, Sue told her mother the doctor and policeman were waiting inside to escort them to the hospital.

'Will you ... would you mind ... coming with me, Mum?' The lip quivered again and Sue broke off abruptly, struggling to keep control. There was something profoundly sad in her isolation. Just when she needed Richard most he was nowhere to be found.

'Of course, I'll come, darling.'

They were all silent as the policewoman steered the car through the evening traffic. Even walking along the familiar corridor towards the Neonatal Unit the figure of the policewoman threw a shroud of unreality around doctor, parent, grandmother. As they neared what had been Peter's room Sue stopped, shrinking back into herself suddenly. The enormity of what lay ahead hit her foursquare.

Roger moved forward taking her arm gently.

'Would you like to go into the Quiet Room first, Sue?' he asked gently.

'Then when you're ready we can bring Peter to you.'

She nodded mutely, tears coursing down her cheeks, stifled sobs convulsing her.

He settled the grieving relatives into the armchairs and went in search of Catherine. She was in the nursery busily tube feeding a very active premature infant who seemed intent on pulling out her tubes.

'Sue with you?' Catherine enquired.

'Uh huh,' Roger's look told her it had been every bit as hard an experience as they had both anticipated.

'How's she taking it?'

'She's letting some of the emotion go now her mother is with her - thankfully. But I don't think Richard's part in this has sunk in yet.'

'Poor woman. Poor woman.' Catherine shook her head sadly.

'What about Wendy?'

'Calmer now. She insisted on staying to see Sue. She has kept herself occupied - stocking trolleys and bays and preparing charts.'

'OK. It's probably only fair that she sees Sue. But not yet I think. Would you like me to take Peter in to the Mum?'

'If you don't mind. I'd like to be here for Wendy - till Sue's ready to see her. I'll just finish this little lady's feed and I'll be with you.'

'Yes, I think we should give them time with the baby first, before they see Wendy.'

'Actually - could I - I'd like to come along myself now just to say how sorry we all are. Would that be OK?'

As Catherine entered, the eyes of all three women flew towards her. Seeing she was empty-handed Sue visibly relaxed her taut shoulders. Words always seemed so inadequate at these times and Catherine simply went straight to her and took both her hands in her own, murmuring something about how losing Peter had profoundly saddened them all. She felt incoherent. The words mattered little to Sue; it was enormously comforting to see the distress of this senior nurse who had loved her baby too and whose life was affected by his passing. Catherine was not regarded as an emotional person in general but she was deeply moved by the death of those infants who had grown enough to become real individuals. Her tears were genuine and for herself as well as for the family. She turned from Sue to clasp Liz Mathieson's hand still clutching a soggy tissue, and tried to convey something of her sympathy.

At that moment Roger appeared carrying Peter wrapped in the hospital's special shawl reserved for these moments. A palpable silence fell on the four women as he entered the room, turning to close the door carefully behind him to give them a moment to prepare themselves. The police constable took several long deep breaths. Catherine and Sue remained transfixed, eyes only on the shawled form. Liz moved closer to throw a protective arm around her daughter's shoulders.

Roger knelt beside Sue and held the baby closer so that she could look before he passed the bundle to her. She shook her head to dislodge the blurring tears. The tiny face looked so dark and wrinkled and somehow different without the tubes and bonnet. Almost as if it wasn't Peter. But it was. Deep inside she knew it was. She reached forward and touched the cold downy cheek. The little head flopped slightly as she turned back the supporting blanket and she recoiled from the gaping mouth.

Deep wracking sobs split the silence as she took the child and held his lifeless body close to her breast, smothering his face with kisses, washing him in her bitter tears. For a long time she remained gripped in this close embrace, lost to all except the excess of her grief. Liz cried unashamedly with her, feeling an added depth of sorrow in her own powerlessness to ease the hurt. Catherine and Roger stood back a few paces, she fighting her own choking tears, he gritting his teeth, forcing himself to watch the harrowing tableau before him for the first sign that intervention was needed.

As the sobbing diminished, Sue relaxed her grip and laid Peter down on her knees. In slow motion she unwrapped the baby until he lay in all his nakedness and she could fully absorb his lifelessness. The actions seemed to stay not only her tears but those of the onlookers. All stood reverently looking at the perfect yet unfinished form. Sue's fingers caressed his head, his trunk, his arms, his legs wonderingly as if she must savour every inch of him during these precious minutes. Roger looked across at Catherine, a brief nod in the direction of Constable Celia Thomas indicating that she too could leave the mother and grandmother alone in their goodbyes. The two women engrossed in the baby scarcely noticed their withdrawal.

When they judged the moment had come to move the process forward Catherine returned to the Quiet Room. She found Sue curled up in the chair crooning gently to the baby once more swaddled in the shawl. The grandmother sat still on the arm of her chair smoothing her hair. The eyes were all dry now and a calm lay over the group. Catherine approached cautiously but firmly.

'Would you like me to take him now? Have you had long enough?'

'No length of time would be long enough.' Sue murmured softly holding the baby tighter for a moment. 'But, yes, you can take him now. Goodbye, my baby. We shall always love you.' The tears welled again as she gazed on the small closed face.

Catherine eased the infant into her own hands and stooped to give Sue a quick hug before she left the room.

'I'll be back shortly.'

At the end of the corridor she handed the body to the waiting staff nurse before returning to Sue and her mother.

'Sue, I want to tell you a bit more about this evening. There's someone else who very much wants to see you.'

Sue was attentive.

'It was Wendy who was looking after Peter tonight when ... when it happened. She feels very badly that she left Richard on his own with Peter. But she did it for the best of reasons. We all appreciate that it's hard for parents to be constantly watched when they're trying to relate to their babies. So it was quite understandable that Richard wanted to be on his own with Peter. D'you see? I know you've been very close to Wendy all along. She's still here. She'd really like to speak to you now. Would that be all right?'

'Of course. I'd like to see her anyway - thank her for all her help.'

Wendy was ashen faced when she entered the Quiet Room with her senior colleague. She hadn't dared contemplate what this moment would be like. If Sue had refused to see her she knew she would have to accept it but there was so much she wanted to convey.

For a second the two women looked at each other. Then as Wendy moved hesitantly forward Sue sprang to her feet and the next moment they were weeping quietly together arms wrapped around each other in mutual comfort and support.

'Oh Sue, I'm so sorry ... so very, very sorry.'

'I know. You loved him too ... I wanted to thank you ... for everything. You've been wonderful. So kind. You've helped us so much.'

'I don't think I shall ever ... forgive myself for leaving them alone ... tonight. I'm so sorry.'

'I'm sure it wasn't your fault. I don't understand what happened - with Richard, I mean. But I know you wouldn't have done anything that wasn't in Peter's best interest. So, don't punish yourself - really, you mustn't. It wasn't your fault. You've been really good to us. After all, it was you, wasn't it? - it was you who gave me the courage to insist our baby was a special person - deserved our best efforts. Deserved to be given the chance.'

'He was a special person.'

'Can you bear to tell me - about what happened? I'd like to hear - you know - how Peter was - everything.'

Wendy looked around at Catherine.

'Is it OK to talk about it? With the police, I mean?'

'I'll check, but I think so.'

They checked. It was deemed acceptable for Wendy to tell the mother the details as she had experienced them. Be careful not to add her own speculations. Wendy tried as well as she could in the face of her own horror to describe Peter's last hours. Sue kept shaking her head, bewildered by Richard's apparent actions, so out of keeping with her knowledge of the man she had known and loved for so many years. If only he would return and they could hear from him what was in his mind. She was sure he would be able to clear up this mystery, if only he could be found.

The night seemed endless. It was painful to leave the hospital now Sue knew there was no reason to return. Every mile that distanced her from Peter tore at her heart. There was no possibility of sleep until Richard returned although she insisted her mother go to lie down. First though she must phone home to explain why she wouldn't be returning to her own bed that night. Dozing in the chair meant so many cruel awakenings as the fierce pain hit her anew each time. Instead she busied herself clearing out the sideboard which had been needing attention for so long. Periodically she heard the crackle of the police walkie talkie and the dull murmur as the waiting constable replied to the incoming messages. It helped her to ply him with cups of tea although she found nothing had any taste for her.

It was not until 4.43pm the following afternoon that there were any new developments. The fresh-faced young policeman sent to sit out the next shift answered the door to the Inspector himself. A muttered conversation took place and Inspector Crammond was removing his hat and entering the Flanaghan's house. Sue was sitting slumped in the chair, exhaustion having overtaken her fierce desire to stay awake until Richard reappeared. Her mother was upstairs having a short nap, her own relief at her daughter's brief respite enabling her to let go of enough tension to sleep fitfully for a short time. Michael Crammond had brought a policewoman along too and she was despatched to waken the grandmother first before they entered the living room.

Liz Mathieson's heart beat erratically as she startled awake to the insistent voice of this strange young woman. It was bizarre. Their normal humdrum lives had turned upside down - they had become surreal caricatures. Policemen wandering around the house. Strange coded messages being exchanged. Much more alien than her favourite TV programmes about the police force. It was decidedly more uncomfortable being involved in these dramas than she had ever imagined and privacy was more precious than she had consciously accepted. She irritably straightened her clothes and smoothed her ruffled hair.

'I'm afraid there's been a development.' Rita Brown's clipped expression sounded so formal.

Liz, still gathering her waking wits, shook her head to bring her more sharply into focus.

'A development?' she repeated vaguely.

'Your son-in-law has been found.'

'Well, thank goodness for that. Now we can get this business sorted out.' Liz shrugged herself off of the bed and reached for her bag. A quick comb would make her feel less exposed to these strangers who prowled into people's bedrooms and used odd phrases.

'It's not quite as straightforward as that, I'm afraid.' Something in the policewoman's voice stopped her in mid reach. She turned slowly to look directly at her. Waiting.

'I'm sorry, but his body was recovered from the river about half an hour ago.'

Liz simply stared. She must be having a nightmare. First Peter. Now Richard. Had the world suddenly gone mad? No words would come from her open mouth as she sat, fingers clenching the sides of the bed.

'He was found in his car in the river at Ninemilend.' Rita tried to soften the information but there was no easy way to give these facts.

Suddenly Liz was sufficiently awake to register something of the implications.

'Sue - his wife - does Sue know?'

'No, not yet. We wanted you to be there for her. So the Inspector wanted you to know first.'

'I must go to her. Oh, my poor baby. Oh, what's to become of her?' her voice became a wail.

Rita kept her own tones calm and even. An hysterical mother she did not need.

'Mrs Flanaghan is asleep in the living room. Inspector Crammond has come himself to break the news to her but he'd like you there with him. Would you like to have a cup of tea before we wake your daughter. Or anything ... stronger ... perhaps?'

Liz shook herself. It seemed so incongruous to be talking about making tea when a great yawning chasm waited to swallow up her daughter. The British panacea for all ills - a cup of tea. But oddly - yes, it might help. In spite of murder - of death - she wanted a cup of tea. Curious. Incomprehensible. But it might help steady her. For the ordeal ahead.

They walked stealthily downstairs to the kitchen. Liz felt a continuing sense of unreality as she set about filling the kettle, brewing the tea, pouring three steaming mugfuls. The Inspector seemed to need the comforting liquid too, she noted vaguely. They talked in low tones as they regrouped as a team steeling themselves for what lay ahead. Liz's instinct was to leave Sue to wake naturally, but a lifelong deference to authority made her put the pressures on the Inspector's time above the needs of her family. Perhaps it was a compromise to sip the scalding tea slowly and spend time cradling the warmth in her hands.

She knelt beside the sleeping form and paused, looking down at the pale face, deep lines etched into its corners. Shaking her head at the cruelty that dealt another mortal blow to this creature who was so dear to her, she sighed deeply. Sue's sleep was clearly light for at the first touch she sprang up, blinking rapidly as she re-entered the wakened world.

'Oh, Mum. You all right?'

'Darling, the Inspector is here to see you. He has news ... it's ... it's Richard.'

Sue's eyes were wide as she looked from her mother's stumbling hesitation to the stolid form of the policeman behind her. Her fingers plucked nervously at her throat and lips as she waited for enlightenment. Something prevented her from verbalising her question. Michael Crammond had lost count of the number of times he'd had to break bad news. but no amount of practice softened the trauma.

'I'm so sorry, Mrs Flanaghan. We've found your husband's car. My men found it - about half an hour ago. In the river.'

Her eyes were great pools of blackness as she stared unflinchingly at him.

'And ...?'

'I'm afraid a body answering your husband's description was found - inside the car.'

She just sat staring at him, unmoving, unseeing.

'Richard's ... d ... dead?' she shook her head slowly back and forth denying her words as she spoke them. 'No. He can't be. He can't be!'

'I'm afraid so, ma'am. I'm very, very sorry.'

'An accident?' Her slow speech sounded as if she were drugged.

'We don't know at the moment. We are investigating a number of possibilities.' He looked down at her with great compassion. Did she suspect? Was she remembering the events of the previous day in the Neonatal Unit or had this second tragedy wiped them out of her mind temporarily. Time enough for the full horror to hit her.

'I'm sorry to have to mention this, ma'am, but I'm afraid we shall need someone from the family to identify the body. I wondered if perhaps - Mr Flanaghan's father?'

'Do they know?' Her wild look was curiously at variance with her dull voice.

'Not yet, no. We had to inform you first. But one of my men will go round to tell your parents-in-law.'

'I don't think - Richard's father- he's not up to ... that. I'll do it. I need to see ...'

The Inspector looked doubtful.

'Oh Sue, no. Not you, my darling.' Her mother was tearfully protesting, clasping and unclasping the hand she had been clutching throughout.

Sue stared down at her as if at a stranger.

'Why not, mother? I've lost my daughter, my baby and now my husband. Why not go the whole hog - identify his body too?' Her voice was stoney, expressionless and her mother wondered fleetingly if the shock had turned her mind.

'Don't you think ... his parents ...?' Her protest was feeble but she had to make an effort.

'Would **you** want to identify **me**?' Sue's voice struck an icy blast around Liz's heart.

She shook her head mutely and shrank away as Sue rose from her chair.

'I'll get my coat.'

'Inspector, can't we do something?' Liz pleaded.

'I'm afraid not. I'm sorry. Believe me - I understand how you feel. But she's the next of kin. It's her right to do it - if that's what she wants. I'd prefer it was the father. But - we can't go against her wishes.' He was sympathetic. He had a daughter about the same age. But he knew that children grew up and made their own decisions.

The cold calm which held Sue in its grip remained until the moment that the mortuary attendant turned back the sheet. The hours lying in the river had distorted his features but it was unmistakably Richard. She fainted into merciful oblivion.

It was not until the following morning that any light could be thrown on events in spite of the best efforts of Inspector Crammond's team of diligent officers. Understanding came in the form of an envelope addressed to Mrs Richard Flanaghan. When she picked it up Sue felt a wave of nausea sweep over her. She clutched at the doorway to prevent herself from falling. The handwriting was Richard's. It had taken two days to travel nowhere. Sue sank into the chair and with leaden fingers tore open the seal.

My darling Sue,
By the time you read this you will know what I have done. I can only hope that one day you will find it in your heart to forgive me.

I cannot face the prospect of watching you killing yourself caring for a deformed and disabled child for the rest of your life. The decision to continue treating Peter was too hard for me to take. I tried to tell you how I felt but you were so insistent that he should live that I think you couldn't hear.

Briony's death was devastating. But death is understandable and time does help us to cope eventually even if it doesn't ever really heal. Peter would have had a living death. We should have been grieving for him all the time, grieving for the perfect child he might have been. And there would be the relentless crippling slog. All day, every day, year in year out for the rest of our lives. And you would have borne the brunt of that. We should have had no time for each other or for Victoria. I couldn't let you take that burden on. I love you too much to stand by and see it happen.

I wonder if you have any idea how much I love you. I have resented having to share you even with the children. You mean everything to me. And it's because of my great love that I have to do this thing. Helping Peter to die will be necessary to save you from killing yourself caring for him. I'm not sure yet just how I'll do it but it will be quick and painless.

I'll make sure he doesn't suffer or linger. Always remember that I loved him too. But I loved you more.

Ending my own life will save you from the publicity and me from seeing the look in your eyes when you find out about Peter. I suspect it will take time for you to understand that I did it for you. I cannot bear to face a time when you might withdraw from me. It is better this way. And I've worked out how I'll do that bit. I am posting this letter second class to ensure I go through with it today. My problem will be getting access to Peter without the nurses in attendance. But because of the letter, I shall think of a way.

Please give Victoria a big hug from her Daddy and in time tell her how much she meant to me. I hope one day she will understand too. I want her to have my collection of books when she grows up. Reading to her all these nights has helped me to capture childhood wonders I never knew. I owe that to her.

I wanted so much to say a proper goodbye but I couldn't. I should have broken down and it would all have been in vain. Leaving you is the hardest thing I have ever done - loving you the best thing in my whole life. Never forget that, my dearest girl.

Try not to be sad. Your parents will help you when I'm not there; they are strong. Make a new life for yourself and Victoria. One day be happy again.

But always remember I am yours for ever, in life and in death.

Nothing can change that now.

With my everlasting love,

Richard.

Without a word Sue rose, handed her mother the letter, and walked as if in a dream out of the room and upstairs to her bedroom. The look on her face forbade Liz to follow. She shuddered, fearful again for her daughter's sanity. The frozen facade Sue had erected around herself since the experience in the mortuary kept her at arms length. She dimly appreciated that this double tragedy had struck deeper than she could feel, but the mother in her wanted to comfort and strengthen. It was profoundly painful to have Sue totally beyond her reach.

With a deep sigh she turned to the letter. Her free hand flew to cover her mouth as she realized with a shock that it came from Richard. Slowly with dawning horror she took in the enormity of the situation. It hadn't been an accident. Richard had planned the whole thing. How could he have chosen such an appalling series of events for her beloved daughter? She crumpled into a weeping heap pounding the arm of the chair in her anger. Upstairs Sue lay stonily staring at the ceiling all emotion frozen. All hope gone.

CHAPTER 10

Life Goes On

It was a double funeral. The tiny white coffin lay beside the dark mahogany, a single rose on each. Dark blood red for Richard. Pale lemon yellow for Peter. As the cortege glided slowly to the church, Sue kept her eyes rigidly on the road. If she looked into the hearse in front she would see again Richard's dead bloated face, Peter's gaping mouth.

She had judged Victoria too young to experience this day and packed her off to a neighbour. Her own parents accompanied her in the foremost car. She knew, from the frequent nose blowing and surreptitious dabbing at her eyes, that her mother was struggling. Her father was simply lost for words and sat very upright in front of her, endlessly turning his hands one inside another. Richard's parents and his brother's family followed in the second car. Sue felt a brief pang - his mother might feel usurped. She had borne him, raised him amd now at his death a new woman who had been part of only a quarter of his life took precedence. She must say something, do something - make her feel she had a special place today.

The long line of cars in the road near the church surprised her. Were they all curious to know how she would bear this final farewell? Some would be friends - people who genuinely cared - but so many? They crawled to a standstill at the church door. She wanted to stay in the darkness within and not face all those eyes. Why didn't people realize it was a sacred moment, intensely private?

The solemn strains of Elgar filled the building as she took her place at the head of the line of mourners. She wished she could hide behind a thick black veil as the royal family did on these occasions. Instead she adjusted her wide-brimmed black hat and smoothed the folds of the new black cashmere coat and drew herself up to her full height. It was a long and lonely walk behind the coffins. She concentrated on staying in time with the music.

The Reverend Mr Simon Monsdale had been very kind. He had come round to the house and talked wisely about being at peace and the comfort of the gospel and even about suicide. Now he spoke kindly about Richard - the man, the husband, the father, the son, the brother, the teacher, the colleague, the friend. He even said nice things about the baby none of them knew. The choice of hymns had been hers but when it came to singing them she was overcome with such emotion that she had to clench her teeth and force herself to think of what she would cook for Victoria's tea tomorrow.

'Yea though I walk in death's dark vale ...'
Yet will I fear none ill:
For thou art with me ...

But he wasn't - Richard wasn't with her. Concentrate on the humdrum. That way you remained dry eyed and in control. Cottage pie might be good - easy and quick, one of Victoria's favourites. Saute the meat and onions. Lots of seasoning. Nice and crispy on the top.

Sue found herself hoping that she didn't need to blow her nose. People might think she was crying if they saw so much as the edge of a handkerchief. If she started she would never stop and there was far too much to be done. Besides, she wanted to be dignified - for Richard's sake. He would have been proud of her.

The reading brought the memories flooding back. Perhaps it had been a mistake to choose something with quite such poignant associations. It was one of their favourite passages - 1 Corinthians 13. All about love. Love - a much more meaningful word than the old rendering 'charity'. But they had always liked the majesty of the King James Version. Just substituted the word love. Then it was just right - right for how they felt.

'Love suffereth long and is kind; love envieth not ...'

Their love had been like that. They had always cared about what the other wanted, needed.

'Love ... beareth all things, believeth all things, hopeth all things, endureth all things.'

How could she endure this thing? Without his love?
'Love never faileth ...'

No, in his own way he hadn't failed her. Richard had allowed his love to take him to death. He had given his life for her peace. If only he had realized - it wasn't what she had wanted. If only he had talked to her about what she really wanted - and really heard her. Without him life was so empty. She would never understand why.

'For now we see through a glass darkly; but then face to face; now I know in part; but then shall I know even as I also am known.'

She devoutly hoped that then - that promised future time - she would understand what now seemed so incomprehensible.

'And now abideth faith, hope, love, these three; but the greatest of these is love.'

As the reading closed she jerked herself back to the present. Who had designed things so that those most closely involved stood nearest to the coffin? In a kinder world they'd have the family at the back. Slip in last - unseen. Slip away before anyone could speak to them. Away into that black world without Richard - without Peter.

It was nearly over.

One more hymn.
'Take my life, and let it be
 Consecrated, Lord, to thee.'

His too, Lord. Accept his life - given for me.

'Take my will, and make it thine;
 It shall be no longer mine.

Richard had overridden her will - he'd made the decision. The wrong decision.

'Take my love; my Lord, I pour
 At thy feet its treasure-store.
 Take myself, and I will be
 Ever, only, all for thee.'

Far too hurtful. Everything hurt now. Like a great open raw wound.

Think of something else. Apricot mousse. Yes, Victoria liked making that. And it slid down easily when you had no appetite.

The grimmest moment came when the two coffins were lowered into the gaping hole - Richard's first then Peter's. When she'd told Mr Monsdale about her dislike of that moment he had tentatively mentioned cremation but she was adamant that they should be buried. When she and Richard had talked about their wishes - about their funerals - they'd agreed it would be a burial. They'd even joked about it - about who would go first. It had seemed so far away. As the brass plaque passed before her eyes and she briefly registered in capital letters RICHARD ALEXANDER FLANAGHAN she forced herself to look up and beyond to the outline of the city and to think of all the thousands of people milling around there completely unaware and unmoved by the catastrophe that had befallen her. Dimly she saw out of the corner of her eye the tiny white coffin with its single yellow rose being lowered after the dark one - deep down, far from sight, taking her heart out of reach of any more pain.

The minister intoned the bit about the sure and certain hope of the resurrection. Then the final prayer. She wished she had something, someone to lean on. She kept her eyes open lest she fall into the hole too. And when it was all over, and Simon Monsdale had gripped her elbow firmly and wished her Godspeed, instead of moving forward to look down into that deep darkness, Sue moved away. She kept her eyes down ostensibly looking at the rows of wreaths lining the drive of the cemetry. They had already arranged that Richard's brother would gather in the cards so she could acknowledge people's kindness. She didn't need to worry about those details. She would just walk steadily across to the car and get to the hotel for all the condolences and then it would all be over.

Two figures detached themselves from the crowd. The first was Inspector Crammond, somehow less awesome in civilian clothes. He took her hand in both his big ones and told her how sorry he was. He wouldn't come to the hotel, work to get back too but thanks for the kind invitation. The second figure was small and neat and all in black. Sue scarcely recognized the red blotched face of Sister Wendy Greenaway but instantly her heart went out to the nurse in her obvious distress. They held one other silently for a long moment. Wendy tried to voice the sympathy she felt, through her sobs. She ended with a self reproachful, 'I'm not very good at these things'.

'It was good of you to come,' Sue's frozen calm unnerved Wendy. 'Richard would have appreciated it. I'm sure he deliberately chose to have you care for Peter - at the end.'

Wendy's chin trembled as she shook her head wordlessly.

'You'll come to the hotel?' The invitation was mechanical but Wendy knew it was sincerely meant. She was enormously impressed by this young woman's control in the face of the utter devastation she must be experiencing. She strongly suspected Sue was still at the stage of being numb and the necessity to organise things and perform certain functions was carrying her through. It would be later on when the enforced activity of the funeral was over and life settled down again that the reality would really hit her. Then there'd be the empty chair, the quiet house, the absence everywhere. But Wendy was on duty in a short while and must get back.

'Could I come to see you - perhaps - in a while? Would you ... mind?'

'Yes, please do. I haven't decided what I'm going to do yet. But if I'm still - still living here - yes, do come.' It was disconcerting to have the right words uttered in such a flat voice. Wendy realized something of the strain of holding herself together that Sue must be experiencing. She made her excuses and slipped away.

Back in the Neonatal Unit she steeled herself to leave the changing room. Roger and Catherine had been enormously kind and supportive but she had felt the embarrassment and discomfort of other staff acutely. They were unsure how to treat her. They seemed to be avoiding her. A bit like being bereaved. People didn't know what to say, kept away in case they hurt you. They knew she was attending the funeral today. They'd be curious to know how it had gone, how she had felt. She just didn't want to talk about it. What she really wanted was to hide herself far away in the privacy of her own rooms, snuggle under the duvet and howl like a baby. Catherine had suggested she change her off duty so she would go straight home but she hadn't wanted to make a commotion, draw attention to herself. So here she was, red-rimmed eyes and pale face singling her out, but otherwise part of the usual team.

Tom Faithful was walking down the corridor as she emerged into the brightly lit Unit. To her surprise he smiled cautiously and said, 'Oh, hi. I think you were very brave to go. I hate the funerals myself. Bring up all sorts of buried emotional baggage.' She was touched by his brusque attempt to comfort and smiled warmly back thanking him as she moved on.

Since the death of baby Peter, Catherine had made concerted efforts to keep Jo Manson away from Wendy. Wendy was certainly not robust enough to take anything like hostility at the moment. However, Jo was herself aghast at what had happened. She could instantly feel for her colleague being an unwitting accomplice in something so alien to her beliefs. She bitterly regretted her own earlier aggression. Made it so hard to reach out and offer comfort. Catherine's intervention felt like a personal criticism - perhaps it was. And it made her feel even more guilty. Not a pleasant feeling.

But she felt a desperate need to speak to Wendy, to make some reparation for the harm she had caused. This was something too deep for her to allow her stubborn pride to stand in the way. She watched for Wendy's return. When she saw the pale face and red eyes, she slipped out of an adjacent room to touch her senior colleague briefly on the arm.

'I'm so very sorry - about what happened. You didn't deserve that. You're one of the best sisters I've ever worked with. I couldn't believe it should happen - to you - you of all people. It was dreadful - such bad luck that it had to be you.'

Tears welled in Wendy's eyes at this unexpected tribute and laid her own hand over Jo's responsively with a choked, 'Thanks, that's kind.'

'And I'm sorry - sorry I was so beastly ...'

'It's OK - I understand. No hard feelings.'

At that moment a shrill ringing of the phone shattered the quiet of the corridor. Wendy reached for the receiver beside her. Triplets at 26 weeks in labour ward. Membranes ruptured, six centimetres dilated. Could someone go down - like now. Ira was bleeped. The whole team swung into motion moving incubators, re-allocating equipment, running drips, preparing sheafs of paperwork. Wendy was swept along with the automatic tide, each member confidently, quietly preparing for another three admissions. She took her usual place in the order of things and the pain of bereavement, of guilt, of bewilderment, receded for the remainder of her shift.

216

It was 11 o'clock that night when she entered her dark empty flat. Physical exhaustion compounded the emotional drain. She turned up the gas fire for comfort. Beside the lamp was a card, a dark background framing a single flickering candle on the front. Inside she had written an apology to Sue Flanaghan. But something had stopped her from taking it today. She could always post it. For a long moment she looked down at the neat precise handwriting. Then with a deep sigh she tore the card into small shreds and consigned it to the wastebin.